797,885 Books
are available to read at

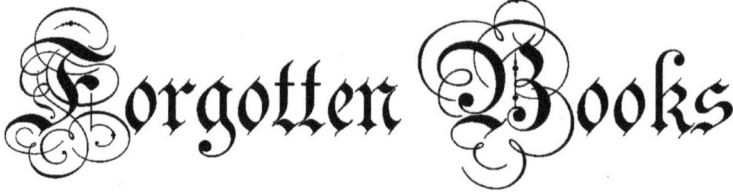

www.ForgottenBooks.com

Forgotten Books' App
Available for mobile, tablet & eReader

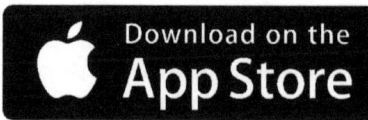

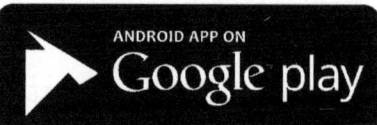

ISBN 978-1-332-23122-5
PIBN 10301703

This book is a reproduction of an important historical work. Forgotten Books uses state-of-the-art technology to digitally reconstruct the work, preserving the original format whilst repairing imperfections present in the aged copy. In rare cases, an imperfection in the original, such as a blemish or missing page, may be replicated in our edition. We do, however, repair the vast majority of imperfections successfully; any imperfections that remain are intentionally left to preserve the state of such historical works.

Forgotten Books is a registered trademark of FB &c Ltd.
Copyright © 2017 FB &c Ltd.
FB &c Ltd, Dalton House, 60 Windsor Avenue, London, SW19 2RR.
Company number 08720141. Registered in England and Wales.

For support please visit www.forgottenbooks.com

1 MONTH OF
FREE
READING

at
www.ForgottenBooks.com

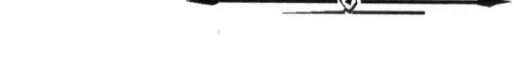

By purchasing this book you are eligible for one month membership to ForgottenBooks.com, giving you unlimited access to our entire collection of over 700,000 titles via our web site and mobile apps.

To claim your free month visit:
www.forgottenbooks.com/free301703

* Offer is valid for 45 days from date of purchase. Terms and conditions apply.

English
Français
Deutsche
Italiano
Español
Português

www.forgottenbooks.com

Mythology Photography **Fiction** Fishing Christianity **Art** Cooking Essays Buddhism Freemasonry Medicine **Biology** Music **Ancient Egypt** Evolution Carpentry Physics Dance Geology **Mathematics** Fitness Shakespeare **Folklore** Yoga Marketing **Confidence** Immortality Biographies Poetry **Psychology** Witchcraft Electronics Chemistry History **Law** Accounting **Philosophy** Anthropology Alchemy Drama Quantum Mechanics Atheism Sexual Health **Ancient History Entrepreneurship** Languages Sport Paleontology Needlework Islam **Metaphysics** Investment Archaeology Parenting Statistics Criminology **Motivational**

of experiment by summing up the objections put forward to them, and to any general adoption of dietaries containing the low level of protein he advocates :

1. The method of basing the protein requirements of the body on the average amount of nitrogen eliminated in the urine gives too low a result for the protein metabolism per kilo of body weight.

2. The very great variations recorded for the digestibility and absorption of protein from identical diets for the individual members of his second group—men of the hospital corps—can either be explained on the basis of malnutrition of the intestinal epithelium, the result of a diet poor in protein, or by failure of the men to collect all the fæces passed each day, so that the total amount included in the analyses was too low. For several reasons we believe the latter to be the more likely explanation. If this should be the explanation, it must throw a certain amount of doubt on the collection of the daily urine for the five months during which this experiment was carried out. Any loss of urine would mean a seemingly lower level of nitrogenous metabolism than was actually the case. It is well known how difficult it is to save all the excretions, except where the most rigid precautions are taken. In the work in India we found it absolutely necessary to confine prisoners under observation to solitary cells, in order to insure the complete collection of the urine and fæces. This criticism would not apply to Chittenden's first and third groups of subjects, who were educated men, and who would fully understand the importance of saving the excreta in full.

3. Whilst one feels bound to accept the figures stated for the daily intake of nitrogen in the dietaries published throughout Chittenden's book, at the same time one cannot help feeling that they would have been much more satisfactory if the nitrogen of those dietaries had been computed from analyses of the dry food materials used, before being cooked, instead of being estimated by means of factors for the percentage of nitrogen in cooked food. The percentage of moisture in any cooked food may vary very considerably from day to day ; this would be specially marked with the more or less vegetarian types of diet Chittenden was compelled to have recourse to in order to keep down the protein content.

Apart from these technical objections which could be easily overcome, there has been considerable mass of criticism levelled at Chittenden's results, and the more remote effects of dietaries low in protein. Hutchison* summarizes some of these, and Crichton-Browne† discusses many others in detail :

1. While a low standard of protein intake may be adopted with apparent impunity for considerable periods, it does not follow that it can safely be pursued indefinitely. Excess of protein is regarded as a margin of safety in increasing the general tone of the system and the resistance to disease. Just as chronic excesses in diet are slow in exacting their penalties, so a subliminal diet may also be tardy in manifesting its untoward effects.

It is generally recognized that abrupt changes in the daily food are very liable to produce gastro-intestinal trouble and failure in health. It is quite possible that radical changes, even when gradually introduced, may have ill-effects of an insidious nature long before there is any obvious breakdown in health.

2. Existence at the lower limits of protein metabolism undoubtedly results in a wasting of the nitrogenous tissues and fluids of the body during every special call or demand for increased effort. This disintegrated tissue may take weeks to replace, and thus convalescence from illness may be prolonged and recovery rendered incomplete.

3. The effects of a diminished protein intake on the race is of far greater importance than on the individual. The experiences gained in India are specially interesting from this point of view, and will be fully discussed presently. Suffice it at present to say, that those people whose dietary affords a low level of protein metabolism are, so far as our knowledge goes, of poor physique, wanting in stamina, and lacking in the manly quantities that are essential in commanding and maintaining the respect of the more virile races.

4. Chittenden's claim, that the elimination of crystalline nitrogenous bodies through the kidneys places upon these organs an unnecessary burden, which is liable to endanger their integrity, and possibly result in serious injury, in so far as it applies to the ordinary accepted standard, cannot be substantiated, and is opposed to universal experience.

Many other points might be raised, some of which we shall discuss in detail later. One very important subject is the bearing of a low protein dietary on the susceptibility to disease. We have

* Hutchison. " Food and the Principles of Dietetics," p. 24.
† Sir J. Crichton-Browne, " Parsimony in Nutrition," 1909

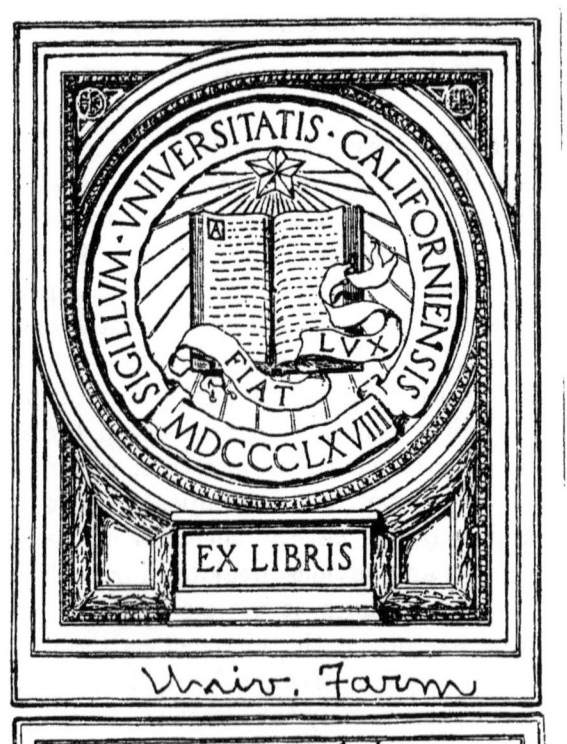

Univ. Farm

QP141
M2

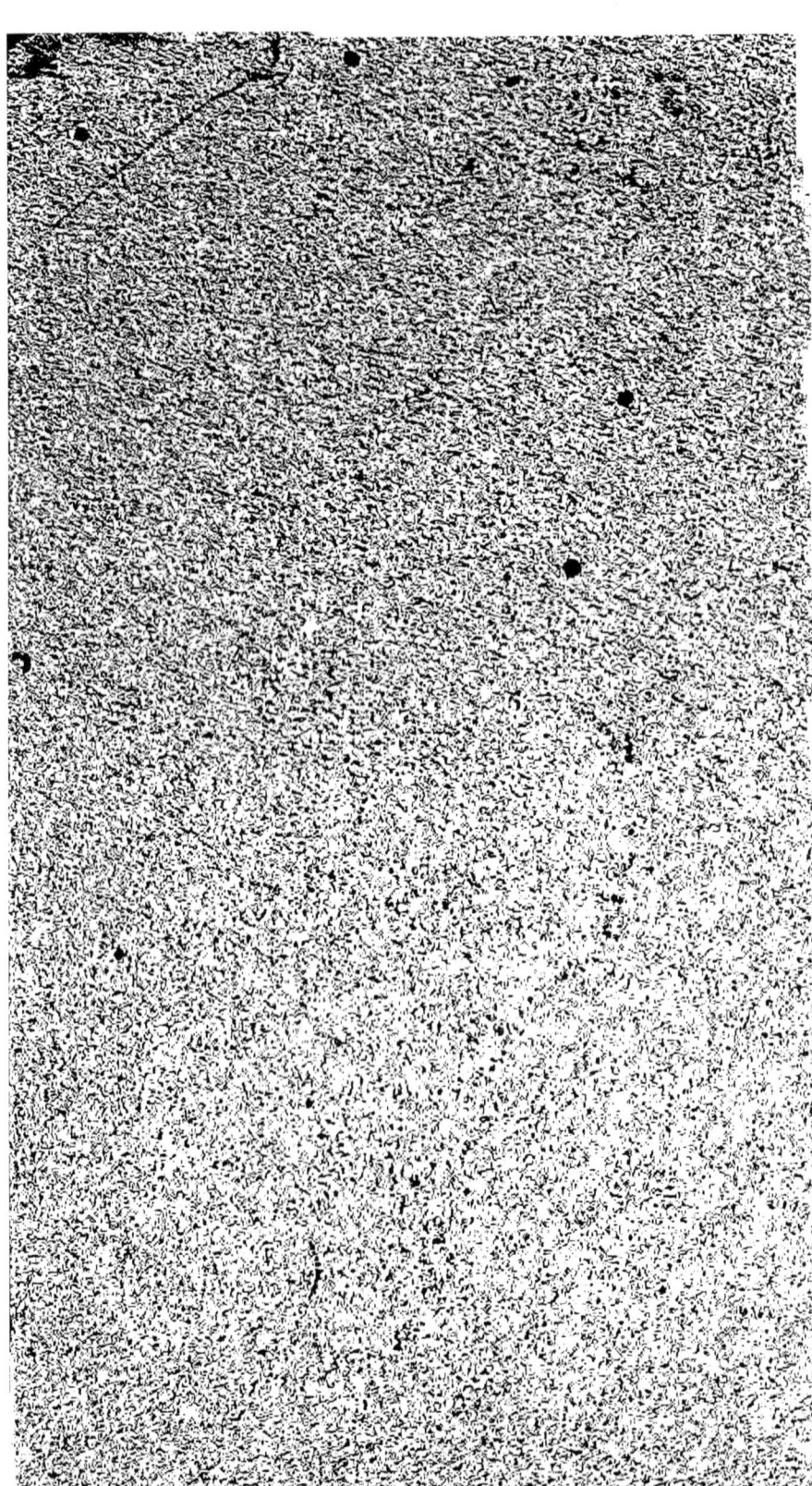

THE PROTEIN ELEMENT IN NUTRITION

INTERNATIONAL MEDICAL MONOGRAPHS

General Editors { LEONARD HILL, M.B., F.R.S.
WILLIAM BULLOCH, M.D.

THE VOLUMES ALREADY PUBLISHED OR IN PREPARATION ARE:

THE MECHANICAL FACTORS OF DIGESTION. By WALTER B. CANNON, A.M., M.D., George Higginson Professor of Physiology, Harvard University. [*Ready.*]

SYPHILIS: FROM THE MODERN STANDPOINT. By JAMES MACINTOSH, M.D., Grocers' Research Scholar; and PAUL FILDES, M.D., B.C., Assistant Bacteriologist to the London Hospital. [*Ready.*]

BLOOD-VESSEL SURGERY AND ITS APPLICATIONS. By CHARLES CLAUDE GUTHRIE, M.D., Ph.D., Professor of Physiology and Pharmacology, University of Pittsburgh, etc. [*Ready.*]

CAISSON SICKNESS AND THE PHYSIOLOGY OF WORK IN COMPRESSED AIR. By LEONARD HILL, M.B., F.R.S., Lecturer on Physiology, London Hospital [*Ready.*]

LEAD POISONING AND LEAD ABSORPTION. By THOMAS LEGGE, M.D., D.P.H., H.M. Medical Inspector of Factories, etc.; and KENNETH W. GOADBY, D.P.H., Pathologist and Lecturer on Bacteriology, National Dental Hospital. [*Ready.*]

THE PROTEIN ELEMENT IN NUTRITION. By Major D. McCAY, M.B., B.Ch., B.A.O., M.R.C.P., I.M.S., Professor of Physiology, Medical College, Calcutta, etc. [*Ready*

THE CARRIER PROBLEM IN INFECTIOUS DISEASES. By J. C. LEDINGHAM, D.Sc., M.B., M.A., Chief Bacteriologist, Lister Institute of Preventive Medicine, London; and J. A. ARKWRIGHT, M.A., M.D., M.R.C.P., Lister Institute of Preventive Medicine, London. [*Ready.*]

SHOCK: The Pathological Physiology of Some Modes of Dying. By YANDELL HENDERSON, Ph.D., Professor of Physiology, Yale University.

DIABETES. By J. J. R. MACLEOD, Professor of Physiology, Western Reserve Medical College, Cleveland, U.S.A.

A Descriptive Circular of the Series will be sent free on application to the Publishers:

LONDON: EDWARD ARNOLD
NEW YORK: LONGMANS, GREEN & CO.

INTERNATIONAL MEDICAL MONOGRAPHS

General Editors { LEONARD HILL, M.B., F.R.S.
WILLIAM BULLOCH, M.D.

THE PROTEIN ELEMENT IN NUTRITION

BY

MAJOR D. McCAY,
M.B., B.Ch., B.A.O., M.R.C.P., I.M.S.
PROFESSOR OF PHYSIOLOGY, MEDICAL COLLEGE, CALCUTTA

ILLUSTRATED

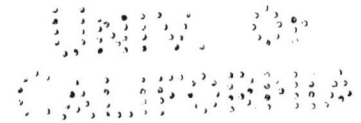

LONDON
EDWARD ARNOLD
NEW YORK: LONGMANS, GREEN & CO
1912

[*All rights reserved*]

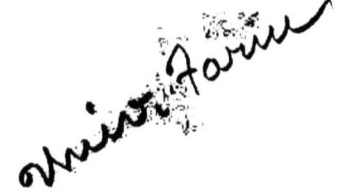

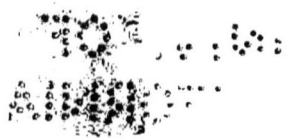

GENERAL EDITORS' PREFACE

THE Editors hope to issue in this series of International Medical Monographs contributions to the domain of the Medical Sciences on subjects of immediate interest, made by first-hand authorities who have been engaged in extending the confines of knowledge. Readers who seek to follow the rapid progress made in some new phase of investigation will find herein accurate information acquired from the consultation of the leading authorities of Europe and America, and illuminated by the researches and considered opinions of the authors.

Amidst the press and rush of modern research, and the multitude of papers published in many tongues, it is necessary to find men of proved merit and ripe experience, who will winnow the wheat from the chaff, and give us the present knowledge of their own subjects in a duly balanced, concise, and accurate form.

Major McCay deals with a subject of fundamental importance —viz, the amount of protein required in nutrition. From prolonged inquiries into the habits and physique of the tribes and races of India, he brings forward a body of evidence which proves that a high protein ratio is necessary in child life to produce a virile and active race of men. Major McCay has had splendid opportunities in the material afforded him by the prison dietaries of India, and he has utilized these to the fullest advantage. His final conclusions are in opposition to those of Chittenden, and demand the closest attention of all, and particularly of those who have to deal with dietaries for the young in schools and institutions.

LEONARD HILL.
WILLIAM BULLOCH.

September, 1912.

280288

AUTHOR'S PREFACE

THE object with which the following pages have been written is to present to the reader a broad view of the subject of nutrition in the light which recent investigations have shed on the problems connected therewith.

Since the publication of the volumes dealing with Chittenden's views on the protein requirements of the body, a very considerable amount of investigation has been quietly going on. Sufficient time has now elapsed, since his first onslaught on the generally accepted opinions held with regard to the level of nitrogenous interchange within the body necessary for the maintenance of a healthy man of average weight and doing a moderate amount of work in health and in a state of efficiency, to permit of definite conclusions being arrived at.

It is meet, therefore, that the stage now arrived at in the determination of the ideal form of the dietary of mankind should be placed on record. Such a record, the author hopes, will be found in the matter set forth under the following chapters.

In the present volume the author has made use of the observations and investigations of a great many of the more important recent publications on the subject, and has attempted to show that the weight of evidence is entirely against the great reduction of the protein content and caloric value of the dietaries of mankind so strongly advocated by Chittenden.

Recent investigations by different research workers have shown that it is possible to reduce very considerably the quantity of protein necessary to maintain an animal in nitrogenous equilibrium, when the particular nitrogenous compounds required by that animal only are given in the food. In fact, at the present time, no one denies the feasibility of maintaining either man or animals in a condition of nitrogenous equilibrium on quantities of protein very much below the standards set up by the old masters in the science of nutrition.

If we knew exactly how much, and what particular nitrogen compounds the body requires in each specific state of nutrition, it is rational to expect that it would be possible to maintain the body in health, vigour, and efficiency on quantities of protein very much less than those hitherto considered necessary; but, as we do not know what form of nitrogen combination nor how much of any particular unit is required in the different states of bodily nutrition, it is surely only rational that, in order to insure a sufficiency of those elements absolutely essential, a liberal standard of dietary should be recommended. The work of Leonard Hill and Flack on flours, and the researches carried out on the production of beri-beri by feeding animals on rice deprived of certain of its outer layers, show how important certain minute constituents of the food may be.

It seems, therefore, only reasonable to lay down such a standard of protein in the feeding of man as will at least give to the body the opportunity of obtaining the particular combinations it requires in any given state of nutrition.

This deduction is fully borne out by a careful consideration of the information available from dietary studies carried out in many different countries, and particularly by the investigations made in India to determine the effects of different degrees of protein interchange on several tribes and races living under exactly the same conditions, except as regards diet. An absolutely dispassionate survey of the physical development and general capabilities of the races and people of India points undoubtedly to the conclusion that, other factors being eliminated, those who obtain a liberal supply of absorbable protein in their daily food are superior in every respect to those whose dietaries exhibit any marked degree of lowering of the average protein standard.

The general conclusion arrived at, from a broad consideration of all the facts available in the present state of our knowledge, is that the views held by the older writers on nutrition are sounder and more in accord with the findings of careful scientific study than are those of the newer school. Voit, who may be taken as a distinguished representative of the former, stands to-day absolutely vindicated; whilst the earnest plea put forward by Chittenden, for a lowering of the protein and caloric value of dietaries by large amounts, cannot be regarded as longer possible, in the light of the accumulated evidence of the ill-effects that follow in the train of chronic underfeeding.

The photographs, illustrating, so far as it is possible to do so, the physique of the different races and tribes investigated, have been very carefully selected as being as nearly as possible typical of the average development met with.

The author tenders his grateful thanks to all those whose works have been of assistance in the argument set forth; wherever possible full acknowledgment has been made in the text. He wishes particularly to thank his assistants in the laboratory, without whose willing co-operation much of the work herein recorded would have been impossible of performance.

D. McCAY.

PHYSIOLOGICAL DEPARTMENT,
  MEDICAL COLLEGE,
    CALCUTTA.
      July, 1912.

CONTENTS

	PAGES
CHAPTER I.—INTRODUCTION	1—22
The importance of protein	1
Advances in our knowledge of the changes taking place during digestion and assimilation of protein	2
End-products of protein hydrolysis	5
The importance of certain necessary end-products in nutrition	6
The necessity of a liberal degree of choice	10
The significance of the denitrification of proteins	12
Schryver's investigations	13
Folin's views on the significance of urinary creatinine and neutral sulphur	15
Later workers on the excretion of creatinine: Van Hoogenhuyze, Verploegh, Paton, Dorner, and Cathcart	17
Mellanby's study of creatinine excretion	17
Schaffer's ,, ,, ,,	17
Levene and Kristeller's investigations	18
Conclusions arrived at with regard to the significance of urinary creatinine	20

CHAPTER II.—THE FOOD OF MANKIND	23—35
The functions of food	23
The great variations in the food of mankind	23
Widespread striving after a mixed form of alimentation	24
Dr. Harry Campbell on the evolution of man's diet	26
His conclusions	30
The chemical composition of European and Indian food materials	31
Heat values of Indian food materials	32
The digestibility and absorbability of foodstuffs	33
Results obtained in Europe and America summarized	34

CHAPTER III.—TROPICAL FOOD MATERIALS AND THEIR DIGESTIBILITY	36—66
Peculiarity of tropical food materials	36
Rice as a food	37
Deficiency in protein	37
Its bulkiness	38
Inferiority of its protein absorption	39
Wheat as a food	42
Protein absorption of good wheat	43
,, ,, of inferior wheat	43
Effects of modern methods of milling	45
The demand for "standard bread"	46
Effects of bleaching	47
,, of adding "improvers"	48

ix

CONTENTS

CHAPTER III.—TROPICAL FOOD MATERIALS AND THEIR DIGESTIBILITY—*Continued*

	PAGES
Relative values in nutrition of white bread, standard bread, and wholemeal bread	50
Conclusions arrived at	51
Maize as a food	52
Protein content and protein absorption	53
Its suitability as a food	54
Barley as a food	54
Protein content and protein absorption	55
Juar as a food	55
Protein content and protein absorption	55
Bajra as a food	55
Protein content and protein absorption	55
Foodstuffs derived from the Leguminoseæ	57
Chemical composition	57
Their importance in the East	58
Work done on protein absorbability	59
Effects of bulk on protein absorption	60
Percentage absorption of the protein of the different legumes	62
Summary of results obtained for the coefficients of the digestibility of tropical food materials	65

CHAPTER IV.—THE PROTEIN METABOLISM OF MANKIND 67—95

Scientific study of dietetics	67
Importance of Chittenden's work	68
Dietary standards, methods of arriving at	68
Generally accepted standards	69
Benedict's estimates of average food consumption	70
Selection of average dietaries in Europe and America	70
Caloric values of army rations in peace and war	71
Atwater's standards	71
Tropical dietaries : Oshima's researches	72
Rice not the principal food material of the tropics	73
Dietary studies in Japan	74
Values of army ration of different nations	74
Dietary of jinricksha man of Japan	74
Effects of alteration in the Japanese Navy dietary	76
Dietary studies in India	76
First study : Students and servants of medical college	76
Bengali and Japanese contrasted	77
Bengali and Chittenden's deductions	77
Second study : Two medical assistants of medical college	78
Third study : Diet scales of different classes of Bengalis	78
Preference for a mixed type of dietary	80
Chittenden's misconception of Bengali's diet discussed : his criticisms answered	81
Chittenden's experiment on six assistants examined : his figures corrected	83
Ordinary Bengali diet not ill-balanced	85
Fourth study : Residential colleges : students' dietaries	85
Fifth study : Dietaries of hill-tribes of Bengal : Bhutias, Sikhimese, and Nepalese	86
Nitrogenous metabolism per kilo of body weight	87
Sixth study : Dietaries of aborigines of Chota Nagpur	88
The meat-eating Todas and salt	88
Nitrogenous metabolism of aborigines	89
Seventh study : Dietaries of the fighting castes of India	89
The foodstuffs of the Sikh	90

CONTENTS

CHAPTER IV.—THE PROTEIN METABOLISM OF MANKIND—*Continued*

PAGES

Nitrogenous metabolism of the Sikh - - - 91
Dietary of the Sikh soldier - - - - - 91
Sikhs not vegetarians - - - - - 91
Eighth study: Composition of Bengali and European mother's milk contrasted - - - - - - 92
Bengali mother's milk deficient both in quality and quantity 93
Average weight of new-born European and Indian infant - 94
Suggested influence of diet on the composition of Indian mother's milk - - - - - - 94
Effects of defective nutrition on the Indian infant - - 94

CHAPTER V.—THE PROTEIN REQUIREMENTS OF MANKIND 96—121

Dietaries considered from standpoint of protein element and caloric value - - - - - - - - 96
Loss of potential energy owing to intestinal fermentation - - 97
The nitrogen of the fæces a true measure of the nitrogen lost to the body - - - - - - - - 99
The protein requirements of the body - - - - 100
  Evidence afforded by the average consumption of mankind - 100
    Chittenden's criticism of this evidence - - - 101
      Crichton-Browne on Chittenden's objections - - 102
      Hutchison's opinion - - - - 102
      Sir William Roberts's opinion - - - - 102
  Evidence afforded by deductions from Folin's observations on urinary creatinine - - - - - 103
  Evidence afforded by a study of the conditions that obtain during starvation - - - - - 104
  The lower limits of nitrogenous equilibrium approximately determined - - - - - - 106
  The lower limits not the most advantageous - - 107
  The increased demand for protein during severe muscular exertion - - - - - - 107
    Paton's investigations and his conclusions - - - 108
    The rôle of protein in muscle work discussed - - 109
      Stewart's opinion - - - - 110
      What the ordinary level of protein interchange really amounts to - - - - - 112
The only way of arriving at the true protein needs of the body - 113
Results obtained from man as to the effects of diets poor in protein - - - - - - - 113
  Different observations summarized - - - - 114
  Chittenden's unique investigations - - - - 114
    The long experiment on himself - - - 114
      Points of interest referred to - - - 115
    His three groups of subjects - - - - 116
      Points of interest referred to - - - 116
  Chittenden's conclusions as to the protein requirements of the body - - - - - - 118
  Chittenden corroborated by:
    Caspari and Glassner - - - - - 118
    Hamill and Schryver - - - - - 118
    The teeming millions of Bengal - - - 118
  Chittenden's most recent work on the degree of protein metabolism exhibited by students - - - 118
    The conclusion drawn from his findings - - - 119
    His work on students adversely criticized - - 119
    His figures corrected and shown to disprove the view he advocates - - - - - 121

CONTENTS

CHAPTER VI.—THE MERITS AND DEMERITS OF DIETARIES POOR IN PROTEIN - 122—148

Chittenden's beliefs regarding danger of excessive protein	122
Foundations for such beliefs not considered valid	123
Criticisms by Hutchison, v. Noorden, and others	123
Chittenden's three groups of experiments, conditions observed, results seemingly obtained, discussed	124
Benedict's critical examination of Chittenden's experiments on soldiers of the Hospital Corps	124
Benedict's criticisms elaborated and discussed	125
The causes of Chittenden's discordant results examined	128
Conclusions arrived at	129
Chittenden's studies with eight athletes	130
Significance of their loss in body weight	131
Regretful absence of controls	131
Objections to and criticisms of Chittenden's experiments and deductions therefrom summarized	132
Other criticisms of a more general nature summarized	133
Nietzsche on the effects of a rice dietary	134
Mullick on the medical aspects of student life in Calcutta	135
Evidence afforded by the dietaries of local and convict prisons in England	135
Dunlop's work for the Prison Commission of Scotland	136
French prison dietaries	136
Other lines of evidence bearing on the effects of dietaries poor in protein:	
Darwin's observations on miners in Chili	137
Livingstone's observations on tribes of Central Africa	137
Zieman's study of coloured races in Africa	137
Irving Fisher's tests of no scientific value	138
Intercollegiate tests in Calcutta and deductions therefrom	138
Evidence afforded by the negro, poor white, and Italian labourer	139
Evidence afforded by the successful races of mankind	140
Experiments on animals:	
Munk, Rosenheim, Hagemann, and Jägerroos	140
Chittenden's experiments on six dogs	140
His work and findings unfavourably criticized	141
Further criticisms	142
Evidence afforded by the feeding of swine on a low and high protein dietary respectively	143
Similar experiments on cows	144
General summary of the evidence adduced	145
Doubts strengthened by a consideration of the caloric values of diets	146
Benedict's observations on Fletcher	146
Heat value of diet of soldiers insufficient	147
Most probable explanation of discrepancy	148

CHAPTER VII.—THE EFFECTS OF A LOW PROTEIN DIETARY IN THE TROPICS - 149—178

Orme on the effeminacy of the inhabitants of Indostan	149
The cause of this effeminacy—a rice diet	150
Scrafton on the effects of a rice diet	150
Cambridge ,, ,, ,,	151
Strachey's opinion	151
The temptation to follow Chittenden's lead	152
Regretful resistance after a study of the results accompanying a low protein intake	153
Macaulay on the characteristics of the Bengali	154
Strachey's comments thereon	154

CONTENTS

Chapter VII.—THE EFFECTS OF A LOW PROTEIN DIETARY IN THE TROPICS—*Continued*

	PAGES
Brahmin proverb exemplifying the effects of diets deficient in protein	155
Facts bearing on the conditions that obtain with the Bengali rice dietary	155
1. The evidence afforded by a study of the urine and blood	156
Tables contrasting the composition of the urine and blood of Europeans and Bengalis	156
Differences examined and significance discussed	157
Deductions drawn and conclusions arrived at	159
2. The evidence afforded by contrasting the physical development of Bengali and Eurasian students living under identical conditions, but on different dietaries	160
The dietaries of the two classes of students	161
Results: Bengali students	162
Eurasian students	162
Their significance in estimating the merits or demerits of diets low and relatively high in protein respectively	163
3. The evidence afforded by a study of the physique, endurance, capabilities of work, and expectation of life in the Bengali	164
(a) Body weight of Bengali shows a low average	164
(b) Height: comparatively tall	165
(c) Chest girth well below European average	165
(d) Physical endurance very deficient	165
(e) Capabilities of work	166
(f) Expectation of life at different ages	167
Mortality rates favourable to Mohammedans as compared with Hindus	167
Evidence collected from insurance companies	168
An actuary's opinion	168
Dr. Adrian Caddy's valuable data	168
Dr. Caddy's results summarized	169
Conclusions arrived at	171
4. The evidence afforded by the resisting power to disease and infection	171
No evidence that an ordinary diet throws any strain on the kidneys	172
Strong evidence that diets deficient in protein are accompanied by malnutrition of renal epithelium	172
Incidence of renal disease in the Bengali	173
Major Rogers's analysis of post-mortem records	173
Resisting power of low protein feeders to acute infections very low	175
Granular kidney and atheroma	177

Chapter VIII.—THE EFFECTS OF THE LEVEL OF PROTEIN METABOLISM ON THE PHYSIQUE AND GENERAL EFFICIENCY OF DIFFERENT TROPICAL TRIBES AND RACES — 179—210

Other factors besides diet as the cause of defective development	179
Chittenden's explanation not valid	179
Dr. Kellogg's criticisms	180
The causes put forward by Kellogg eliminated	180
Peoples of Behar, Lower Bengal, Orissa, and Eastern Bengal contrasted	181
The true facts regarding the level of nutrition and the fighting instinct	182
The evidence obtained from an examination of the dietaries of the hill tribes of Bengal and their physical development	184
The level of protein metabolism and the conclusion arrived at as to its effects	187

CONTENTS

CHAPTER VIII.—THE EFFECTS OF THE LEVEL OF PROTEIN METABOLISM ON THE PHYSIQUE AND GENERAL EFFICIENCY OF DIFFERENT TROPICAL TRIBES AND RACES—*Continued*

	PAGES
The evidence afforded by a study of the races of the Gangetic Plain	188
The different physical types	189
Rajputs: Eastern and Western	191
Western, superior as soldiers	192
Effects of differences in diet	192
Physical development of Rajputs	193
Dogras: Rajput Highlanders	193
Growth of caste system	193
Characteristics of the Dogras	194
Effects of diet on physique	195
Diet and foodstuffs of Dogras	195
Different classes of Dogras: Effects of diet on:	
(a) Dogra Brahmins	196
(b) Dogra Rajput:	
i. Mian Rajput	196
ii. Rana and Thakur classes	197
iii. Rajputs of the Plains	197
iv. Lower classes of Dogras	197
Summary of available information on the effects of differences in diet	197
Diet and physique of Dogra recruits	198
Jats: Eastern and Western Jats	199
Differences in diet and religion	199
The Jat Sikh: His diet	200
His physique	201
Summary of evidence collected	201
The Sikh: Characteristics	202
Effects of Sikhism	203
Effects of diet	204
Physical development	204
Summary and conclusions	205
The Pathan: His food	205
Characteristics	205
Physique	205
Summary of the importance of a high level of protein metabolism	206
Other Indian frontier tribes illustrate the importance of protein, such as the Afridis, Waziris, Bajouris, Baluchis, and many others	206
Further evidence afforded by the investigations of the Committee on the physiological effects of food, training, and clothing on the soldier	207
Lieut.-Colonel Melville's opinion	207
Aron's experiments on the effects of a restricted diet on growing dogs	208
His conclusions	208
Their close correspondence with the conditions that obtain in the rice-eating Bengali and Ooriya	208
The influence of certain substances, present in the food in small quantities, on nutrition	208
Hill and Flack's researches	209
Funk's isolation of beri-beri vitamine	209
Experiments to show that the absence of these bodies from the food will not explain the poor physique of the Bengali	210
Points raised, discussed	210
INDEX	211

LIST OF PLATES

		FACING PAGE
I. (a) Bengali; (b) Ooriyas		58
II. (a) A Group of Rice-Eating Ooriya Children; (b) A Group of Better-Class Ooriyas		86
III. (a) Tibetan Bhutia; (b) Nepalese or Bhotanese Bhutia		108
IV. Sikhim Bhutias		156
V. Nepalese Coolies from Nepal		172
VI. (a) Tibetan Woman from Gyantze; (b) Tibetan Woman from Lhassa; (c) Nepalese Woman from Nepal		186
VII. (a) Punjabi Mohammedan; (b) Dogra		194
VIII. (a) Rajput; (b) Sikh; (c) Pathan		204
Photograph of Rice-Eating Bengali Coolies	page	177

THE PROTEIN ELEMENT IN NUTRITION

CHAPTER I

INTRODUCTION

"The life-processes consist in the metabolism of the proteins."—VERWORN.

THE important part played by the complex body protein and its allied nitrogenous compounds is acknowledged by all students of nutrition.

As a food material it is the one constituent that is indispensable; it is the only substance of the three main classes of proximate principles that is absolutely essential for the carrying out of those vital phenomena whose aggregate may be considered to represent the processes of life.

The more important tissues of both animal and vegetable life consist largely of this protein material, and it is in connection with the changes protein undergoes within the living organism—the chemical changes by which the protein of the food is prepared for absorption and incorporation into the bioplasm, the changes which it undergoes while it shares in the life of the tissues, and, finally, those by which it is broken down again into waste products and eliminated from the body—it is in connection with these that much of the interest in the subject centres. It is but natural, therefore, that the chemistry of metabolic processes should have attracted the attention of large numbers of investigators. The result of this has been that the literature of the subject has already attained enormous proportions.

Progress, despite the vigorous activity displayed by a yearly increasing number of workers in physiological chemistry, has not been very conspicuous. In recent years, however, owing to the introduction of new methods of attacking the problems connected with protein metabolism, remarkable advances have been recorded, particularly with regard to the nature and chemical constitution of the proteins and their cleavage products.

By the process of breaking down the large complex protein molecule into smaller, less complex bodies or units, and by the method of building together again such cleavage products into substances in many respects similar to the ordinary nitrogenous compounds, much light has been thrown on the nature of proteins and on the arrangement of their molecules. The main results of these investigations are to show that the protein molecule is built up of a series of units or organic radicles—the amino-acids—which form the basis of their composition. These amino-acids may be looked upon as the building-stones or units of the protein molecule, and it is in virtue of their presence that the protein molecule possesses the peculiar property of building itself up into bodies of high molecular weights. The results obtained by means of hydrolytic agents on the different proteins show definitely that they are all composed of the same units; in some cases certain organic radicles or building-stones are missing, and in some cases certain of these building-stones are greatly in excess.

The importance of these discoveries can only be grasped when it is borne in mind that the old views regarding the changes in protein material during digestion are rapidly undergoing modification. The fact that proteins are an essential part of the food of all animals was interpreted to mean that no synthesis of proteins occurred in the animal body, so that all proteins in existence must necessarily be the products of the vegetable cell. In fact, on this basis a fundamental distinction was drawn between the nutrition of plants and animals. The long dominant doctrine of Liebig, that plants in the main live without protein food, and are able to construct their own proteins for themselves, whilst animals have to find their proteins ready-made in their food and are unable to build them up, no longer holds good. The further the study of the nature and constitution of the different proteins advanced, the more clearly evident did it appear that animal and plant proteins were different in type; the investigations in the science of serology would even make it practically certain that the protein of one species of animal is quite different from that of any other species, and even the proteins of the different organs of animals of the same species differ from one another.

At present our conception of the effects of the digestive enzymes is very different from what was held to be the case even a few years ago. The indiffusible colloid substance, protein, was formerly supposed to be modified in such a manner by the hydrolyzing agencies of the intestinal tract that, as a final product, peptone—a diffusible substance—was formed. The trypsin of the pancreatic juice was known to be able to carry the hydrolysis beyond the stage of peptone, but Kuhne, who first investigated its action, arrived at the conclusion that trypsin was only able to affect half of the protein molecule. It is now known that both pepsin and trypsin can liberate very many of the products of acid proteolysis, and to a great extent destroy the protein character of the substance on which they act. Further, the ferment erepsin of the succus entericus is able to cause a more complete breaking down of the peptones and albumoses that have escaped the action of pepsin and trypsin, so that most observers are unanimous in thinking that the hydrolysis of proteins in digestion is complete. In the light of recent work it is evident that the breaking down of the protein molecule of ingested material, due to the action of the digestive enzymes, goes on to the actual splitting up into organic radicles—the amino-acids and other crystalline derivatives. These derivatives of protein digestion—a large number of which have now been isolated and many of them synthesized—resemble in the main the units or building-stones obtained as cleavage products in the acid hydrolysis of proteins *in vitro*. There is experimental proof that the final products of tryptic digestion are able to take the place of protein in the food. Otto Leowi maintained a dog in complete health with an increase in body weight on the products of pancreatic digestion, the chemical observations showing that no protein was present in the food, and that the daily amount of nitrogen metabolized was less than that ingested. Henriques and Hansen have successfully carried out similar experiments on rats, and have confirmed these results. From the building-stones or cleavage products of protein digestion the body is, therefore, capable of building up its bioplasm, and of making good the wear and tear of everyday life; in doing so, in all probability, different sets of units or amino-acids are made use of in the formation of the many different types of nitrogenous material required by the several tissues of the body. That is, the material out of which all proteins in the body are made is not protein in any form, but the organic radicles derived from proteins by hydrolysis, which in different combinations and in different proportions are found in the proteins of the different tissues, these different combinations and proportions conferring on the nitrogenous material of the several organs and tissues a specific character.

But while the cleavage products of the intestinal digestion of proteins are able to maintain an animal in nitrogenous equilibrium, those formed by the hydrolytic action of mineral acids are quite unable to do so; animals fed on these substances live no longer than other animals whose food contained no nitrogenous materials at all. There is therefore some difference in the hydrolytic action of the digestive enzymes as contrasted with that of mineral acids, although the products obtained by the action of these two hydrolyzing agents are to a large extent identical. However, it is evident that the acid breaks up some building-stone or stones which the digestive ferments retain, and which are absolutely essential in the synthesis and nutrition of the bioplasm. What the nature of those organic radicles may be whose presence are of such importance in the assimilation of the products of tryptic digestion, at present it is impossible to say. It may be, as Leathes suggests, that there is some kind of linkage between certain groups in the protein molecules which is not broken down by the digestive enzymes, but is in acid hydrolysis. When this coupling is destroyed, it is impossible for the cells of the body to make use of these groups, and successfully resynthesize them into materials necessary for the nutrition of their bioplasm.

The study, therefore, of the intermediate stages in the processes of protein metabolism has opened up a field for research, which has been and is being successfully cultivated. As pointed out above, the researches of Fischer, Kossel, Schutzenberg, and a host of others have thrown a flood of light on the composition of the protein molecules. Protein has been shown to consist of a complicated chain of units capable of being broken down into bodies of gradually decreasing complexity. Thus, the first real decomposition products of acid or enzyme proteolysis are the albumoses which exhibit distinct characteristics, and are easily isolated by precipitation with ammonium sulphate. The next products—the peptones—are less definitely characterized, and are at present identified by one positive reaction—the biuret test. Fischer has applied the term "peptides" to a number of bodies which are derived from peptones, but which no longer give the biuret test.

These peptides contain several molecules of crystalline organic radicles—the amino-acids—and break down into these on further decomposition. Finally, a large number of simple end-products of protein hydrolysis have been discovered, isolated, and, during the last few years, many of them have been synthesized. These bodies have been classified by v. Noorden into the following groups :

    I. Monamido-Acids :
        (*a*) Monobasic—
            Glycocoll, alanine, serine, isoserine, amido-valerianic acid, leucine, tyrosine, and phenylalanine.
        (*b*) Dibasic—
            Aspartic acid and glutaminic acid.
    II. Diamido-Acids :
        Lysine and arginine.
    III. Indol- and Skatol-Producing Group :
        Tryptophane, skatolamino-acetic acid, or indo-lamino-propionic acid.
    IV. The Pyrrol Group :
        Pyrrolidine-carboxylic acid.
    V. The Pyrimidine Group :
        Histidine.
    VI. The Carbohydrate Group :
        Glucosamine.
    VII. The Sulphur-Carrying Group :
        Cystine.

The simplest of the amino-acids contain one organic radicle and one basic radicle—the acid character being due to the carboxyl group COOH, and the basic character to the amidogen group NH_2. Amino-acids containing only one amidogen group are classed as "monamino-acids," as $CH_2(NH_2).COOH$, glycocoll, or mono-amido-acetic acid ; others possessing two such basic groups are termed "diamino-acids," as $CH_2(NH_2).(CH_2)_3.CH(NH_2).COOH$, "lysine," or "$a\epsilon$-diamido-caproic acid." In the majority of the amino-acids there is only one carboxyl group, but sometimes there are two or more such groups, and then they are classed as "monobasic," "dibasic," etc. One of the peculiar characteristics of these amino-acids is their power of undergoing conjugation or condensation with one another, or with other organic radicles, to form more complex bodies with high molecular weights. So far, however, all attempts to build up proteins from the amino-acids have failed. Emil Fischer has built up bodies which he calls "polypeptides," by the condensation of glycocoll, leucine, and other amino-acids. It is hoped that the formation of these bodies may be the first step in the process of protein-synthesis.

Another important discovery in connection with the formation of the intermediate products of protein metabolism is that the cells of nearly all the organs of the body have been shown to possess enzymes capable of breaking down the complex protein molecules, and causing disintegration as complete as in the action of the ferments of the intestinal tract. That the breaking down of the nitrogenous tissues begins as a result of the action of these cellular enzymes is most probable, and is supported by the fact that some of the products of protein hydrolysis are found in the bile and urine, having escaped further destructive changes which would have terminated in them being excreted as urea or other nitrogenous constituent of the urine. Glycocoll is an example of one of the products which has escaped this fate ; by its union with cholaic acid it is found in the bile as glycocholic acid, and with benzoic acid it occurs as hippuric acid.

Another property of the cells, again probably the work of an intracellular enzyme, is their power of liberating ammonia from the amino-acids. This power is most marked in the cells of the intestinal mucous membrane and liver, which would explain the fact that the percentage of ammonia in the portal blood is during digestion several times greater than that in the systemic blood. The significance of this power of the cells of the intestinal mucous membrane and liver of denitrifying the hydrolyzed products of protein digestion is not clear ; but it has been explained as being a reaction which, while leaving the non-nitrogenous part of the protein molecule untouched, facilitates the greater part of the nitrogen of the hydrolyzed products of protein digestion in being eliminated in the urine as urea. The speed with which a large part of the nitrogen appears in the urine as urea, following on the ingestion of a protein meal, has been taken as a sign that the body does not require all the nitrogen, and that it must be got rid of before the valuable part of the protein molecules is admitted into the general circulation. This is effected by the denitrifying action of the enzymes of the cells of the intestinal mucosa and liver. The fact that the greater part of the nitrogen of the food is quickly eliminated, and never reaches the tissues of the body at all, suggests at once that the amount of nitrogen provided in ordinary dietaries is too great. This is a subject which will require very careful consideration; at present, all that need be said is that this denitrification has not been proved to apply to all the products of protein digestion. In fact, it is very doubtful if it occurs at all, or at least to any great extent, in those amino-acids or building-stones that are absolutely essential for the nutrition and repair of the bioplasm. It may be that only the ordinary amino-acids, which probably have to be taken in excessive quantities in order that there may be a sufficiency of the more important compounds, undergo denitrification with speedy elimination of their nitrogen as urea in the urine. Thus, tyrosine and phenyl-alanine are said not to increase the output of urea when injected into the blood; and histidine, which contains a nitrogenous group related to one of those found in nucleic acid, does not give up its nitrogen in the form of ammonia. The feeding experiments of Kaufmann and Murlin with gelatin, where, in spite of a very large intake of nitrogen, equilibrium could not be maintained, while great improvement in the conditions occurred when small quantities of aromatic bodies, normally absent from gelatin, were added; the work of Hopkins and Willcock on zein, where marked effects followed the addition of tryptophane to the diet—these and other experiments of a similar nature would appear to show that in a diet it is not so much the actual amount of nitrogen that is of importance, but that the food ingested must contain a sufficient amount of the particular building-stones necessary for growth and repair.

In accordance with this view the work of Michaud is most important, as demonstrating that the intake of nitrogen can be reduced to a minimum, and nitrogenous equilibrium maintained when the food contains nitrogenous compounds in the proportions suited to the animal's requirements; this he effected by feeding animals on the flesh of their own species—a dog on dog's flesh. It is probable that in breast-fed infants the milk presents the necessary ingredients in the proper proportions, so that the hydrolysis of the proteins in the digestive tract, and the subsequent synthesis of the cleavage products into the proteins of the tissue cell, can take place with a minimum amount of waste.

Further, it is known that certain substances formed in certain organs are absolutely necessary in the maintenance of health, as, for instance, the substances elaborated by the suprarenals, thyroid, pituitary body, etc. Adrenalin is derived from an aromatic precursor, and Hopkins believes that the suprarenal requires a constant supply of some one of the aromatic groups of the protein molecule to serve as an indispensable basis for its elaboration. If such a constant supply is not available, as, for instance, in starvation, a precursor would have to be provided by the breaking down of some of the tissues of the body.

In connection with the necessity of the body being provided with the particular combinations of units suited to its needs, it is important to bear in mind that the proteins contained in food— whether animal or vegetable—are different in composition from those found in the tissues of the body. The products obtained from various proteins on hydrolysis show very marked differences in the proportions of the various amino-acids. These differences are well brought out in the table opposite.

It is evident, therefore, that in protein metabolism the body selects the particular combinations it requires, and builds them up into its own peculiar types of nitrogenous matter, and that the type of protein supplied in the food is of little importance, so long as it is capable of furnishing a sufficiency of the particular types of amino-acid needful in the synthesis of tissue proteins. The feeding experiments with gelatin, already referred to, is a good instance of the importance of the presence of special combinations of molecules in the food. The rôle of protein in the diet cannot be undertaken by gelatin because, although gelatin can be broken down into different amino-acids, such as arginine, lysine, histidine, etc., it is unable to provide tyrosine, tryptophane, or cystine, all of which are essential in the synthesis of tissue proteins. The addition of these bodies to a diet of gelatin enhances its value enormously, so that it may even take the place of true protein. Further proof of the power the tissues possess of forming their own particular types of protein, whatever the diet may be, is forthcoming in the experiment of Abderhalden, who bled a horse until a large quantity of the serum-protein was lost. The animal was then fed on gliadine, which contains four times as much glutamic acid as horse's serum-protein ; in spite of the absorption of gliadine the serum-protein of the horse's blood remained the same. The same holds good for the vegetable

Proteins.	Glycine.	Alanine.	Leucine.	Phenyl-Alanine.	Tyrosine.	Serine.	Cystine.	Proline.	Oxypro-line.	Aspartic Acid.	Glutamic Acid.	Trypto-phane.	Arginine.	Lysine.	Histidine.	Ammonia.
Egg-albumin ..	0·00	2·10	6·10	4·40	1·10	..	0·30	2·30	..	1·50	8·00	+	..	..	..	..
Serum-albumin ..	0·00	2·70	20·00	3·10	2·10	0·60	2·50	1·00	..	3·10	7·70	+	..	..	..	..
Lactalbumin ..	0·00	2·50	19·40	2·40	0·90	..	..	4·00	..	1·00	10·10	..	..	..	..	..
Clin from horse's blod ..	0·00	4·19	29·04	4·24	1·33	0·56	0·31	2·34	1·04	4·43	1·73	+	5·42	4·28	10·96	..
Serum-globulin ..	3·50	2·20	18·70	3·80	2·50	..	0·70	2·80	..	2·50	8·50	+	..	..	..	..
Fibrin	3·00	3·60	15·00	2·50	3·50	0·80	1·10	3·60	..	2·00	10·40	+	..	..	..	1·99
Legumin from peas	0·38	2·80	8·00	3·75	1·55	0·53	..	3·22	..	5·30	13·80	+	10·12	4·29	2·42	..
,, from beans	1·00	2·80	8·20	2·00	2·80	..	..	2·30	..	4·00	16·30	..	4·60	5·10	1·10	2·10
Protein from maize	0·30	..	6·20	1·80	3·80	..	..	5·00	..	0·70	12·70	+	7·10	3·00	3·00	3·61
Zein from maize ..	0·00	2·23	18·60	4·87	3·55	0·57	0·45	6·53	..	1·41	18·28	0·00	1·16	0·00	0·43	5·11
Gliadine from wheat	0·02	1·33	5·67	2·35	1·20	0·13	..	7·06	..	0·58	37·33	+	3·16	0·00	0·61	4·87
Hordein from barley	0·00	0·43	5·67	5·03	1·67	..	..	13·73	..	..	36·35	..	2·16	0·00	1·28	1·60
Caseinogen from cow's milk ..	0·00	0·90	10·50	3·20	4·50	0·23	0·06	3·10	0·25	1·20	11·00	1·50	4·84	5·80	2·59	2·50
Gluten from wheat	0·40	0·30	4·10	1·00	1·90	..	..	4·00	..	0·70	24·00	+	4·40	2·20	1·20	0·40
Gelatin	16·50	0·80	2·10	0·40	0·00	0·40	..	5·20	3·00	0·60	0·90	0·00	7·60	2·80	0·40	

protein, zein, experimented with by Hopkins and Willcock. Zein, given in the food, cannot be recovered from the tissues, and in all probability certain of its amino-acids are made use of to build up tissue protein; certain other units, not being of the particular composition required, are rejected and eliminated as waste.

From the standpoint of the synthesis of tissue proteins by selection of those particular amino-acids or units that are suitable, it will be acknowledged that, in the proper nutrition and growth of the nitrogenous tissue, a protein diet in excess of the actual requirements will be necessary, in order that the body tissues may have plenty of choice. This principle would hold good for all proteins, but especially for protein of vegetable origin, for, if the amino-acids formed during digestion are not present at all, or not present in the necessary proportions, and this is all the more likely to be the case with vegetable proteins, then, the suitable groups being relatively scanty, much unsuitable protein will require to be hydrolyzed in order that the proper supply of the essential units may be obtained. In the light of the opinions at present held regarding protein synthesis within the body, these considerations would forcibly combat the view that has been put forward that great benefits would accrue to the economy from dietaries low in protein, unless it could be absolutely insured that the low protein dietary supplied just those particular amino-acids in sufficient quantities which the body required.

The modern views held regarding the substance protein, the changes that are brought about during digestion, its fate after absorption, and the processes by which it is finally broken down into waste products, may now be briefly summarized.

By the united efforts of the three ferments, pepsin, trypsin, and erepsin, the breaking down of the protein molecules during digestion is a far-reaching process, the protein being disintegrated into a series of organic radicals, of which the amino-acids are the most important. These amino-acids may be looked on as the units or building-stones from which the protein molecule is made, the numbers and combinations of these units differing in different proteins, and being by no means the same in the proteins of the food as in the body proteins. During this demolition of the protein molecule into amino-acids, the protein loses but little of its potential energy.

These amino-acids are taken up by the epithelial cells of the intestinal mucous membrane, and whether transformed into the serum-proteins by these cells, or passed on into the blood as amino-acids and other final products of hydrolysis, is, for the present, an open question. The evidence on the whole would make it appear probable that the products of the digestive hydrolysis of proteins enter the blood unchanged, and are taken up by the tissue cells at a rate not appreciably different from the rate at which they are absorbed by the blood from the intestine. In the somewhat analogous condition in plants during germination, proteins, stored as food material in the seed, undergo hydrolytic changes, and circulate in the sap in the form of amino-acids practically identical with those formed during digestion in animals. In the plant nitrogen is supplied to the cells in the form of these cleavage products during the period of active growth, and it is from these that the vegetable proteins are built up.

Whether in the form of synthesized serum-proteins, or, what is more likely, in the form of the unchanged products of digestive hydrolysis, the protein of the food finds its way into the blood. The evidence available at present would point to the conclusion that the amino-acids, on passing through the cells of the intestinal mucous membrane, are to a great extent, robbed of their nitrogen, which is split off from them in the form of ammonia. This ammonia, which Nencki found to be present during digestion up to four times the normal amount in the blood of the portal vein, is converted in the liver into urea and eliminated as such in the urine. This fate, however, only befalls those units or fragments of the protein of the food that are not required for the building up or repair of tissue protein, or that are not required by the body at that particular time. The units that are then in demand, and which may be quite different from those needed for repair at a different period, are made use of by the tissue cells for their growth and nutrition, and for the supply of the necessary complexes of molecules which are broken down during the ordinary disintegration of living tissue ever taking place.

It has been pointed out that this seemingly wasteful method of making use of precious protein material was open to a different interpretation to that which appears on the surface, and to that put forward by the advocates of the superiority of a low protein dietary. Evidence has been adduced to show that unless the proper and suitable building-stones were furnished in the final products of protein digestion, it did not matter to the body how much protein the diet contained; the result would be the same as if no nitrogen were present in the food at all. The necessary building-stones would have to be obtained from the disintegration of the inferior tissues of the body in order that the master tissues should be maintained as long as possible in a state of nutrition and repair. When those particular building-stones are known and can be supplied in the food, it has been found possible to reduce the protein element of the dietary to a minimum. The danger of such a procedure in the general dieting of mankind is made apparent when it is recognized that the particular amino-acids required in any given state of body nutrition cannot possibly be known, and this danger is enhanced by the fact that in the ordinary food materials, particularly in those of vegetable origin, the amino-acids are not present in the proportions (sometimes not present at all) necessary for the building up of tissue protein. It is clear, therefore, that in the selection of a sufficiency of suitable units a great many end-products of protein digestion that are not required will be rejected—their nitrogen split off, and got rid of as urea. In order that the body may receive a sufficiency of the particular units it requires, a good supply of protein in the food is essential, a supply very much greater than what would be necessary if the suitable combinations were offered in the diet.

But while it is true that within a few hours of the ingestion of a protein meal seemingly a large part of its nitrogen is eliminated as urea, it does not necessarily follow that the nitrogen split off is of no service in nutrition. In fact, it is well recognized how very important a part ammonia does play in those pathological conditions where there is an over-production of acids within the body.

In acidosis and acid intoxications it is of the greatest importance that the acids formed should be disposed of in some way without involving any reduction in the alkalescence of the blood. This can be effected by the ammonia derived from protein metabolism, and which is on its way to be changed into urea. Ammonia is, therefore, of considerable interest as one of the chemical defences of the body against disease. By combining with and neutralizing organic acids, sometimes formed in excessive amounts, it permits of their elimination in the urine without depleting the blood of its important bases. However, outside this use in pathological conditions, ammonia would appear to have an important function in the ordinary nutrition of the body. Recent investigations by Schryver have opened up a very interesting line of research, and if his results hold good, they would tend to raise the status of ammonia from its present position, as a mere by-product of little or no importance, to that of one of the most important units in the physiological processes of nutrition.

By means of carefully carried out experiments, he has shown there is no evidence that the products of tryptic digestion as such can circulate in indefinite quantities in the blood-stream, and that there are no such bodies present in the liver. What, then, is their fate after leaving the alimentary tract? Schryver finds that the difference between the total nitrogen and the nitrogen of coagulable albumin is very high in the mucous membrane of the small intestine, a tissue most intimately connected with nitrogenous metabolism. This difference is higher in the carnivora than in the herbivora; it is independent of the state of nutrition, and is the same in fasting as in the fed animal; and, lastly, that the bodies represented by this nitrogen are in a state of loose chemical combination with the bioplasm, such as exists between an enzyme and its substrate. In this state they undergo certain chemical changes like hydrolysis or oxidation; the products of the change would be eliminated and carried in the blood-stream to other parts of the organism, their place being taken by similar bodies, the product of tryptic digestion, which in their turn would undergo a similar series of changes.

The passage of the products of tryptic digestion through the mucous membrane of the intestines would therefore be analogous to a continuous chemical process. The bioplasm acts as an enzyme or collection of enzymes, to specific points of which side-chains are anchored; it always keeps saturated with side-chains, as is shown by the fact that the residual nitrogen is the same during digestion as during a fast.

That this saturation of the bioplasm is automatically maintained, the following considerations would make probable:

Autolysis occurs more rapidly in the liver of a fasting animal than in that of an animal during active digestion; it is inhibited by the action of ammonia and other alkalis, but accelerated by the presence of acids, especially lactic acid. The acceleration due to acids is a function of the absolute quantity of acid present, at least for sulphuric acid. Lastly, the liver eliminates ammonia on treatment with weak alkalis, and more is obtainable from the organ of a well-fed animal than from that of a fasting animal—more also from carnivora than in the case of herbivora.

It is known that during the constant disintegration of living tissue, or autolysis, bodies of an acidic nature are produced—carbonic acid, lactic acid, etc. ; therefore, by applying the above considerations to what is known to occur during digestion and metabolism, it will be evident that, so long as an animal is well nourished, there will be an excess of ammonia present, and the tissues will show no signs of acidity. This excess, however, will gradually disappear if the animal is deprived of food. A stage will soon be reached when the production of acid exceeds the amount of ammonia available for neutralization. Owing to the acidity, autolysis will be set up, and amino-acids will be liberated. These amino-acids would be carried to the alimentary tract, and ammonia would be split off, as in the case of the products of tryptic digestion. This ammonia, by restoring the alkalinity of the liver and tissues, would inhibit the autolytic processes. Degradation of tissue should proceed at a definite uniform rate.

From his results Schryver arrives at the following conclusion : In order to maintain nitrogenous equilibrium, nitrogenous foodstuffs must be ingested in such quantities and in such form that the amount of ammonia produced therefrom in the digestive tract is sufficient to maintain the intracellular alkalinity of the liver, and probably other tissues.

If this view is correct, it would mean that the ammonia split off from the final products of tryptic digestion plays an important rôle in nutrition, as it maintains the general intracellular alkalinity, in the absence of which nitrogenous equilibrium ceases to be longer possible. When the protein offered in the food is deficient in either quantity or quality, the acidic processes generated in the organism set going the autolytic enzymes ; the amino-acids thereby liberated are carried to the side-chains of the bioplasm of the cells of the small intestine, keeping them fully saturated even in starvation, and free ammonia is generated by the hydrolysis or oxidation of those bodies they replace. This ammonia inhibits temporarily the further disintegration of the tissues, and so long as present in sufficient amount would favour anabolism. The anabolism and katabolism of the tissues may therefore be looked on as the result of antagonistic reactions, the balancing of which results in nitrogenous equilibrium.

The only other point it is necessary to refer to in this summary of the intermediate products of nitrogenous metabolism is the importance that has been attached to the constancy in the amount of certain of the waste products that are eliminated in the urine. Folin has shown, and his results have been confirmed by many observers, that the output for the same individual of creatinine and neutral sulphur in the urine is constant, that this output does not alter with the change from a nitrogen-rich to a nitrogen-poor diet, and that the output seems only to vary with the mass of the nitrogenous tissues of the body. (Cathcart, experimenting on himself, found a distinct difference in the output of creatinine whilst fasting and on an ordinary mixed diet.) Folin holds that these substances, creatinine and neutral sulphur, are characteristic of endogenous or tissue metabolism, whilst urea and other nitrogenous constituents, the output of which varies with changes in the composition of the diet, are indicative of an exogenous or intermediate metabolism. From the results obtained for the output of creatinine in the urine—which seem to vary for the same individual under different dietaries from 0·353 to 0·534 gramme, expressed as nitrogen—a whole theory of protein metabolism has been built up, and great importance has been attached to it as affording strong evidence that only very small quantities of nitrogen are necessary to maintain the organism in full bodily vigour—just that amount, in fact, that is required to make good the ravages of endogenous metabolism, of which the constant output of creatinine and neutral sulphur in the urine is in some way a measure. The underlying suggestion is, although Folin himself does not state so, that these two forms of metabolism are absolutely distinct from one another, and that urea is almost, if not entirely, an excretory product of exogenous metabolism.

According to the older views of Liebig and Pflüger, the products of digestion circulate in the blood-stream, or are built up into the bioplasm, the proteins of the blood plasma and lymph forming the source from which the cells derive their supply. All katabolism of protein material must, therefore, be preceded by anabolism. The discovery that a large proportion of the nitrogen of a protein meal appeared in a few hours as urea entailed the belief that the protein absorbed from the food has been very quickly built up into the living protoplasm, only to be accompanied, or immediately succeeded, by a similar degree of katabolism. As this explanation did not appear very probable, in the light of Nencki's finding of a large excess of ammonia in the blood of the portal vein during digestion, this view is not regarded now as sufficient to cover the facts. It is considered much more probable that the ammonia split off from the amino-acids of tryptic digestion is transformed into urea in the liver, and that the nitrogen represented by that urea never reaches the protoplasm of the cells, but is quickly got rid of in the urine.

The constancy in the output of creatinine for each individual has been suggested to mean that this substance is a product of true tissue metabolism; the one factor determining its amount being the weight of the true tissue elements of the body. Further, creatinine has been looked upon to some extent as a measure of the extent of the nitrogenous interchanges within the body; and as the total daily output rarely exceeds 0·6 gramme nitrogen, it has been used as an argument to support the view that only a small amount of protein is needed in the diet. The line of reasoning from this point of view is quite clear. Shortly, it is as follows :

The products of tryptic digestion lose a large proportion of their nitrogen on absorption; this exogenous katabolism appears to have no physiological meaning, and the extent to which it takes place in the ordinary individual on a liberal protein diet no justification. The constant splitting off of nitrogen appears to serve no useful purpose, as the organism can neither use it nor store it up for future use. The carbohydrate moiety of the protein molecule is made use of as a source of body heat and potential energy, but this could easily be replaced by carbohydrates given as such in the daily food. Having the further information that the nitrogenous requirements of the true cellular tissues—as measured by the products of endogenous metabolism—are very small, the question naturally arises, Would it not be greatly to the benefit of the organism to lessen the protein element in the diet to an amount closely approximating that of the true needs of the body ? This question the advocates of a low protein dietary answer in the affirmative. The true answer can only be arrived at by a very careful consideration of the principles involved in all their bearings, and particularly by an investigation to determine the effects of a limited supply of protein in the food on the physical well-being of the individual or of a race.

Since the introduction of Folin's colorimetric method of creatinine estimation, a great amount of research has been carried out on its elimination under various conditions of diet intake and energy output. Van Hoogenhuyze and Verploegh made a large series of experiments to determine the effect of exercise; they arrived at the conclusion that muscular work only produces an increased elimination of creatinine when the body is forced to live at the cost of its own tissues, as in starvation. Noël Paton and Dorner, later also Cathcart, found a relation between the creatinine excreted and the intaken protein.

The most complete study of the subject, however, is by E. Mellanby, and the conclusions he has arrived at are of considerable importance in connection with the views expressed by Folin and others. The broad general conclusions to which Mellanby comes are, that in the formation of creatinine muscle plays a small part, whilst the liver, on the other hand, is intimately connected with the production of creatine and the excretion of creatinine.

He believes the liver to be continuously forming creatinine from substances carried to it by the blood-stream from other organs, that in the developing muscle this creatinine is changed to creatine and stored, while after the muscle has reached a saturation-point creatinine is continuously excreted. Mellanby brings forward a considerable mass of evidence to support his conclusions. The fact that in the chick creatinine is not excreted until a week after hatching, which he shows by analyses to mean that the muscles are not until then saturated with creatine; that there is almost complete absence of creatinine from the urine of young children and also of puppies, lends added support to his findings.

Later, Shaffer, from a careful study of the excretion of creatine and creatinine by normal and pathological subjects, arrives at the conclusion that creatinine is not an index of total endogenous protein katabolism. Subjects of exophthalmic goitre and others, in whom the total endogenous katabolism is probably much increased, excrete very little creatinine. He states that creatinine is derived from, and its amount is an index of, some special process of normal metabolism taking place largely, if not wholly, in the muscles, and upon the intensity of this process appears to depend the muscular efficiency of the individual.

Still more recently Levene and Kristeller undertook a series of investigations as to the rôle of the muscular system in regulating the creatinine output. Observations were made on twenty-four patients affected with disease in which the muscular system was involved. The influence of diet was also studied whenever the creatinine output was found abnormal. Three forms of diet were generally employed: one of low protein content, but containing sufficient calories, the nitrogen intake not exceeding 6 grammes, and the calories reaching 3,000 per day; the second diet of approximately the same calorific value contained milk and eggs, with a nitrogen content of about 10 grammes; and the third, a beef diet, with a nitrogen content of 20 grammes per day. In health these diets should not markedly influence the creatinine output.

A review of the results brings to light the following facts:

In all pathological conditions involving the muscular system the rate of katabolism of ingested creatine is lowered, and part of the ingested substance is removed in the form of creatinine. When there was dissolution of muscular tissue with diminution of muscular activity, the output of creatinine was low and that of creatine high. In some cases the output of both creatine and creatinine was influenced by the protein content of the diet. The findings cannot be interpreted adequately on the basis of any one of the existing views on the mechanism of creatine metabolism. Thus, Shaffer's hypothesis that the extent of creatinine output is determined by muscular efficiency does not harmonize with the observations on progressive muscular atrophy, where there may be an extreme degree of muscular wasting, without any marked alteration of the creatinine output. Folin's theory, which regards the intensity of cellular katabolism as the principal factor in influencing the creatinine output, is not supported by these investigations. Mellanby's view, likewise, is not sufficient to interpret the results obtained. These authors believe that in the regulation of the creatinine output at least two factors are concerned: the formation of the substance, very probably from protein, and its further oxidation. Any disturbance of either may lead to an abnormal output of creatinine.

The constant value in the amount of the creatinine output in normal individuals is explained as being due to a condition of high velocity of creatine combustion in health. The creatinine of the urine only represents a small fraction of the creatine formed in the organism. The uric acid output in the dog appears constant, as in this animal the oxidation of purin derivatives is exceedingly high, so that only a minimal amount escapes in the urine as uric acid. However, as soon as the liver is excluded from the circulation, and the intensity of the purin oxidation is diminished, the uric acid output in the dog begins to show marked variations, influenced by the character of the food. Similarly, the normal creatinine output in conditions of high muscular activity may be explained by a greater power of the organism to oxidize creatine, although creatine production in these conditions probably exceeds the normal limits. They found, for instance, that only 48 per cent. of ingested creatine reappeared in the urine of a patient who was suffering with continuous tremor, whilst in conditions of atrophy or dystrophy practically 90 per cent. escaped oxidation, and was recovered in the urine.

More recently still Krause and Cramer, working on the effects of thyroid feeding, find that on a meat-free diet administration of fresh raw thyroid gland is followed immediately by a marked rise in nitrogen excretion, which persists for several days. This increased nitrogen excretion is accounted for by increased urea elimination, and not by an increase in the creatinine elimination.

Since the effects of thyroid feeding on nitrogen metabolism can be observed in the fasting organism and with a nitrogen-free diet, it would appear that changes in the nitrogen metabolism observed after thyroid administration are due to changes in the tissue or endogenous metabolism.

According to Folin's view, one would expect to find a marked increase in the excretion of such constituents as creatinine and neutral sulphur, which he believes are the end-products of endogenous metabolism. The results show, however, that this is not the case, but that the changes induced in the endogenous metabolism of thyroid feeding result almost exclusively in an increased formation and excretion of urea and ammonia.

In the light of these recent researches on the factors which regulate creatinine metabolism, it is evident that the rate of creatinine elimination is not a function of the intensity of cellular katabolism, and is no measure of the total nitrogenous interchanges taking place within the cells of the different tissues—
i.e., between the protoplasm of those cells and the nutrient

materials of the blood plasma and lymph. It would appear much more probable that the formation of creatine and creatinine represents two phases in the katabolism of one substance, the result of a special process in normal metabolism, as a fall in the creatinine output is usually associated with an increased creatine elimination, and a high protein diet (creatine-free), in some patients is accompanied by a rise in the output of both substances.

It has been shown by Weber that a larger amount of creatinine is to be found in the perfusion fluid when the heart is in action ; whilst, on the other hand, muscular exercise has been confirmed by many observers to cause no rise in the creatinine output. It would, therefore, follow that the creatinine formed in muscle during its activity, and removed from that tissue by the blood is further changed in the organism, only a small fraction of the creatinine of muscle escaping oxidation and appearing in the urine. According to Hoogenhuyze and Verploegh, the power to oxidize creatinine is inherent in all organs.

It is, therefore, still very doubtful what the origin of creatinine in the body is : whether from the nitrogenous products of the daily food, or by some special process of normal metabolism, according to some observers, probably intimately related to changes in muscle. It is still more doubtful what the fairly constant quantity of creatinine eliminated in the urine is significant of. There seems to be a general consensus of opinion that it represents an unoxidized fraction of the whole amount formed in the body. There is very little evidence in the more recent researches supporting Folin's view that it represents endogenous metabolism, or that it can be regarded in any way as a measure of the nitrogenous interchanges of the protoplasmic tissues of the organism. The deductions that have been drawn from his conclusions regarding the origin of creatinine as a product of cellular metabolism can no longer be considered convincing. Thus Folin believes that the constant or endogenous metabolism is largely represented by creatinine, and to a slight extent by uric acid. The deduction from this in Chittenden's words is, considering " these views so admirably worked out by Folin, the question naturally arises, if the real demands of the body for protein food will not be adequately met by the quantity necessary to satisfy the true tissue metabolism." Folin also states in the same connection that only a small amount of protein—namely, that necessary for the endogenous metabolism—

is needed. As it would appear improbable that creatinine originates in the body from the type of endogenous metabolism Folin has created; also, that, even if this were the case, it cannot possibly be a measure of such metabolism, the deduction drawn that, being a small and constant output, therefore only a small and constant supply of protein in the diet to replace the nitrogen represented by its loss is necessary must be fallacious.

It may be concluded, therefore, that, so far as the evidence goes, the output of creatinine in the urine cannot be made use of as evidence to support the arguments of those who consider that the protein requirements of the body would be covered by the presence of a very limited amount of nitrogen in the daily food.

This finishes our summary of the recent advances that have been recorded in the investigations into the intermediate stages of protein metabolism. Beyond a knowledge of certain changes that take place in proteins during the process of digestion, very little accurate information is available. With regard to the series of chemical reactions by which the products of tryptic digestion are made use of by the protoplasm of the cell for its growth, nutrition, and repair, we know practically nothing. Still, a beginning has been made, and enough light has been shed on some of the individual chemical reactions of the body to enable us to look forward with hope and confidence to the future; otherwise, as Verworn puts it, the fact that wherever the gross activities of the body are traced to the activity of the individual cells, we always come upon an unsolved problem might lead us to maintain with Bunge: "All processes in the organism which may be explained mechanically are no more phenomena of life than are the movements of the leaves and branches of a tree that is shaken by the storm, or the movements of the pollen that the wind wafts from the male poplar to the female."

Amongst those things that give promise of hope in the future are the advances that have been made in the conception of the part played by enzyme action in metabolic processes. At present a great variety of chemical reactions within the body are brought about in virtue of the presence of a large group of intracellular enzymes. In addition to the action of the digestive enzymes, which resolve protein, carbohydrates, and fats into their components, many oxidizing enzymes have been found in the various organs and tissues. Instances of these are met with in the group of autolytic enzymes, which are present in the different tissues, and which split proteins into amino-bodies and nitrogenous bases; other examples are guanase of the thymus, adrenals, and pancreas, which converts guanine to xanthine; adenase of the spleen, pancreas, and liver, which converts adenine to hypoxanthine; catalase found in many tissues, and which decomposes peroxides—this has been looked on as the reason why oxidation takes place only in certain tissues, and not in others where it is not required, as, for instance, in the blood. The extension of the conception of the work of enzymes to all phases of metabolic activity has greatly enlarged the outlook, and has brought within measurable bounds the time when it will be possible to explain the causes upon which the chemical activities of the body depend.

REFERENCES

The following works of reference, monographs, and original papers have been consulted and freely made use of in the preparation of the foregoing introduction.

VERWORN : General Physiology. London, 1899.
LEATHES : Problems in Animal Metabolism. London, 1906.
HILL : Recent Advances in Physiology and Bio-Chemistry. London, 1906.
HILL : Further Advances in Physiology. London, 1909.
CHITTENDEN : The Nutrition of Man. London, 1907.
SUTHERLAND : A System of Diets and Dietetics. London, 1908.
SCHÄFER : Textbook of Physiology. London, 1898.
V. NOORDEN : The Physiology of Metabolism. London, 1907.
CATHCART : Protein Metabolism : Journal of Physiology, vol. xxxix., 1909.
MELLANBY : Creatine and Creatinine. Journal of Physiology, vol. xxxvi., 1908.
LEVENE AND KRISTELLER : Factors regulating the Creatinine Output in Man. The American Journal of Physiology, vol. xxiv., 1909.
SHAFFER : The Excretion of Creatinine and Creatine in Health and Disease. The American Journal of Physiology, vol. xxiii., 1908.
SCHRYVER : Studies in the Chemical Dynamics of Animal Nutrition. The Bio-Chemical Journal, vol. i., 1906.
PLIMMER : The Chemical Constitution of the Proteins, part i. London.
KRAUSE AND CRAMER : Proceedings of the Pyhsiological Society, May, 1912.

CHAPTER II

THE FOOD OF MANKIND

THE functions of food are, first, to build up the different tissues of the body, and repair the waste of ordinary wear and tear; secondly, to furnish energy for the production of muscular contraction and other work the body has to perform, and to yield heat for the upkeep of the body temperature.

Foodstuffs may, therefore, be considered from two points of view—viz., their power or capability of forming new tissue and repairing waste—this is a function of the assimilable or available nitrogenous material; its power of yielding energy and heat—this is a function of all the organic elements of the food, protein, carbohydrate, and fat. The food as taken into the body differs very much in its chemical composition from the materials that are utilized in carrying out the above functions, and it is by the processes of digestion that the proximate principles of a diet are split up and rendered easy of absorption into the blood and lymph, and are prepared for assimilation and utilization by the several tissues of the body.

A review of the different foodstuffs entering into the dietaries of mankind reveals a most varied assortment, differing, under the varying conditions of life on the earth, with the seasons, climate, customs, races, and countries. At one extreme, as pure animal feeders, may be taken as examples the Esquimaux and the Indians of the Pampas; whilst at the other extreme, as almost pure vegetarians, may be cited many of the natives of the tropics in the East Indies. It may be accepted, however, that the food of the inhabitants of any particular place depends on local circumstances, and will vary with the food materials available during the different seasons, with the cost, and with the ease with which it can be procured. Thus the Esquimaux live practically of necessity upon raw or partly cooked seal, walrus, and whale; the Fuegians subsist largely on seal and porpoise; and the Indians of the Pampas for many months in the year cannot obtain other food than fish.

It is generally believed that the inhabitants of the tropics, and more particularly, perhaps, the Hindus, are practically pure vegetarians. This is by no means the case. In India and in the torrid zone generally the natives eat largely of cereals, fruit, and vegetables, and many of the poorer classes cannot afford other food; on the other hand, where any form of animal diet is procurable or can be afforded, except the flesh of animals forbidden by religious customs, it is greedily and readily seized on and devoured. Even amongst the so-called vegetarians of India milk and eggs are always allowed; many also eat fish, and some conform their vegetarian principles to the occasional presence of chicken or goat's flesh in their dietaries.

In a densely populated country such as India, the mass of the inhabitants have got to live on the cheapest food procurable, which in a country not yet thoroughly opened up is usually the home-grown products, consisting largely of cereals, fruits, and vegetables. They are vegetarians by force of circumstances only, and readily avail themselves of every opportunity of increasing their assimilable protein intake by the addition of most forms of animal food to their diets. The craving for highly nitrogenous food, and particularly that of an animal nature, was well brought out during some feeding experiments on prisoners in Bengal, when the promise of meat, or the threat of withholding it, was quite sufficient to induce the prisoners to carry out without a murmur whatever duties had been assigned to them. In the less densely populated districts of Bengal, where there is not the same necessity for the extensive cultivation of the land and production of vegetable foodstuffs, animal food of all kinds forms quite a fair proportion of the diet. Thus the aboriginal races inhabiting the hills of Chota Nagpur eat all kinds of flesh, including that of rats, jackals, snakes, lizards, and other animals.

The Hindu cannot, therefore, be accurately described as a vegetarian by instinct. On the average, doubtless, his diet contains considerably less animal matter than the mixed diets that are customary in the temperate zone, but this is entirely due to his inability to obtain the meat he craves for, and not to any subtle promptings of Nature warning him against the evil that may result in a torrid clime from a liberal protein dietary. The fact, indeed, that animal food should be so much desired and, when obtained, so greedily devoured would afford strong evidence that certain "fundamental, instinctive, nutritional demands" have been interfered with by the competition of a dense population, and that the mass of the people are existing in a condition of nitrogen starvation, and require far more assimilable protein than their vegetable dietaries provide.

The same desire for a mixed form of alimentation is met with in all countries and climates. Thus Major Woodruff, Surgeon, U.S.A., writing of the inhabitants of the Philippine Islands, says: "The natives do not eat meat because they cannot get it. They crave it, need it, and eat it when they can." Before the emancipation of the Japanese from the strict tenets of Buddhism, which prohibited the taking of life under any circumstances, even for food, fish had to be allowed, just as is the case amongst the Buddhists in India to-day. Fish not being a prohibited article of diet, according to Japanese ideas anything that could be called "fish," whatever might the stretch of the imagination required to do so, could likewise be eaten. The eating-houses in Japan advertised mountain whale, which really meant venison; so venison may be eaten. The same holds true for the natives of India, from the highest inhabitable ranges of the Himalayas to the plains of the southern parts of Madras. Except amongst certain narrow sects where prejudice is rampant, animal food is partaken of freely where financial conditions do not bar the way; and when cost is an obstacle, it is made use of to as great extent as can be afforded.

Mixed animal and vegetable food may therefore be looked upon as the ordinary type of diet of the great majority of mankind, despite the restrictions of country, climate, or race; indeed, there is distinct evidence of a striving after a mixed form of alimentation in the evolution of man from the earliest geological periods down to the present time. There can be little doubt but that the evolution of man's diet has exerted a very marked influence on the evolution of man himself and on his dissemination over the face of the earth. Buckle affirms that the increasing supply of food, "as wandering tribes advanced from the hunting to the agricultural state, had momentous moral consequences by diminishing dependence on mere chance, and opening the mind to a conception of the stability of events and the laws of Nature; while of all physical agents by which the increase of population is affected, food is the most active and universal. Where the national food is cheap and abundant, population inevitably increases more rapidly than where it is scarce and dear."* With regard to the function of animal food in man's evolution, Crichton-Browne states : " In whatever direction the temper of the mind be bent by animal or vegetable diet, it is clear that animal food has played a decisive part in human evolution, and that the craving for it has largely contributed to the advance of civilization. That craving led to the invention of weapons and traps of many kinds, to the acts of fishing and hunting, to migration, travel, and adventure, to the patient pursuit of the taming and domestication of wild creatures, and to provision for their wants ; and success in the satisfaction of that craving has always been followed by advancement alike in the arts of war and peace. A diet rich in protein makes for physical and mental energy, and it is not vegetable protein—always poor in amount to the bulk of the food eaten, difficult of absorption, and probably of special and, from a nutritive point of view, inferior constitution—but animal protein that is required. It is animal protein that is the true food of the brain and nerves, and hence all the more energetic races of the world and those most distinguished for intellectual capacity have been meat-eaters."

In connection with this most interesting subject, the brilliant work that has been done by Dr. Harry Campbell† in adding to our knowledge of the changes man's diet has undergone from early times is of first importance, and demands careful consideration.

Of the three classes of the mammalia—as regards diet—the frugivora, including such animals as the squirrel, rat, and the monkey, are mixed feeders. Being generally more intelligent than the herbivora, and gifted with considerable prehensile powers, they are able to pick and choose their food, selecting it in its more concentrated forms, such as seeds, nuts, fruits, eggs, small birds, lizards, grubs, and the like. " Man, now essentially a mixed feeder, belongs by virtue of his descent, as might be expected from his high mental and bodily development, to the frugivora."

With regard to the food of evolving man, Campbell points out that " the products of the uncultivated vegetable kingdom are by themselves totally inadequate to supply man's nutritive needs." The fruits and vegetables of the present day are very different from their wild and barely edible representatives of past ages. They in their turn have undergone an evolution no less remark-

* Sir J. Crichton-Browne, " Parsimony in Nutrition," 1908.
† Dr. Harry Campbell, " The Evolution of Man's Diet."

able than that of man, and yet "even now no existing race of man, in spite of the most elaborate methods of preparing and thus increasing the nutritive value of its vegetable food, is capable of subsisting on it alone." Animal food, prior to the period of cibiculture, was accepted in every form procurable. Of course, the choice would be limited to the smaller forms of animal life until such time as evolving man learned to hunt, fish, trap, and fashion weapons.

Three great factors influenced the changes the diet of evolving man has undergone since presimian times. These factors were the kind of food available; the instinctive liking for certain kinds of food, which depended on the richness of the food in nutrient material, its digestibility, and its taste; and, lastly, the ability to secure the desired food. The food of the great apes and the monkeys at the present time consists largely of the more concentrated vegetable substances, with a certain proportion of animal food in addition. That they, like man, are descended from ancestors whose diet was bulky, and was composed mainly of vegetable material, is evidenced by the presence of a large cæcum and the possession of a vermiform appendix. "The diet of primates, as of all highly intelligent animals, is a concentrated diet, consisting of concentrated vegetable foods, and to a less extent of the yet more highly concentrated animal foods."

Dr. Campbell goes on to trace the dietetic career of evolving man from simian times onwards, and shows that it was characterized by three signal advances, each of which greatly augmented the supply of food. He tabulates the following epochs and periods:

1. The precookery epoch—from the ape stage to the invention of cookery.
   - The simian period.
   - The homo-simian period.
   - The early hunting period.

2. The precibicultural cookery epoch—from the invention of cookery to the introduction of agriculture and the breeding of animals for food.

3. The cibiculture epoch—from the time man began to produce his food artificially to the present day.
   - The period of migratory agriculture.
   - The period of stationary agriculture.
     - (Early.)
     - (Late.)

The homo-simian period saw the evolution of ape to man, and his gradual spread from Southern Asia or Northern Africa over the Indo-African continent. As intelligence increased a greater supply of animal food was obtained, so that he became more of a flesh-eater and less herbivorous.

The early hunting period dates from the invention of weapons and devices for hunting and fishing, such as are employed by the representative of the precibicultural epoch at the present time. As he passed through the homo-simian period his diet became more and more of an animal nature, and in the hunting period he developed largely into a carnivorous type. At this stage of evolution, as his skill in hunting increased, man was able to disseminate far and wide over the earth, as he was able to obtain sufficient food by hunting, and from fruits and seeds.

THE PRECIBICULTURAL COOKERY EPOCH.—As soon as evolving man began to apply artificial heat to his vegetable food, he greatly augmented his supply, as by cooking the vegetable cellulose was broken up, and the nutritive materials set free. The effect of the introduction of the art of cookery was that more vegetable food was used than in the early hunting period, until it came to constitute one-half or more of the total diet, as is the case with precibiculturists at the present time. Another effect was the abandoning of, and the corresponding loss of power to digest in the raw state, the less digestible and less palatable kinds of vegetable foods, until he eventually limited himself to the easily-digested kinds only. "The most primitive peoples now living cook their food, and though widely separated both ethnologically and geographically, they employ identical methods of cookery. Thus the aboriginal Australians and Californians, the Bushmen, the Andamanese, and the Ainus, all know how to extract noxious principles from their vegetable foods, and all employ underground ovens." The identity in the methods employed by these peoples would show that they had taken their methods of cookery with them when they first migrated from a common centre. All existing precibiculturists know how to cook with underground ovens, but some of them have not yet attained the level of discovering how to boil water. Such is the case with the Australian aborigines, the Fuegians, and the Bushmen of South Africa.

It is of importance in discussing the food of mankind to take into consideration the food of the existing precibiculturists. There are still many representatives of this epoch of man's evolution—races who neither cultivate the vegetable kingdom nor breed animals for food. Included amongst them are the aboriginal Australians, the Andamanese, the Californian Indians, the Esquimaux, the Bushmen of South Africa, the Veddahs of Ceylon, and the hairy Ainus.

Their dietary consists of—

Animal Food.—Practically every species of animal is acceptable: Worms, scorpions, moths, grasshoppers, sandflies, crickets, locusts, centipedes, caterpillars, grubs, insects and reptiles, white ants, frogs, toads, lizards. Big game forms the chief supply—deer, antelope, elk, lion, and hyæna—though most of these are but seldom procurable. The Esquimaux practically live on the seal, walrus, and whale; and the Fuegians on the seal and porpoise. Fish of all kinds, salmon, shellfish, clams, etc., are all made use of by precibicultural maritime tribes.

Vegetable Foods.—Roots: Root-digging is a most important source of food. Small seeds: It is suggested that the recognition of the high nutritive value of grass seeds led to the cultivation of cereals (wheat, barley, oats, rice, maize, and millets), a step which was in all likelihood a forerunner of civilization. Large seeds and nuts: Acorns, sunflower, cactus, water-melon, and several species of pine and leguminous plants. Fruits: Many varieties of fruits and berries are eaten. Green vegetables: These are chiefly valued for their component salt and water.

Fungi, seaweed, and gum are all made use of.

The precibiculturists store their vegetable foods. He consumes a large part of it in a raw state, while cibiculturists cook nearly all vegetable foods. No existing precibiculturist has learned yet how to extract starch or sugar from his vegetable food materials.

Honey forms a most important item of nutriment, except in the case of the Esquimaux and Fuegians.

THE CIBICULTURAL EPOCH.—"A great step forward was taken when man began to produce food artificially, when, instead of having to search laboriously for fruits, roots, and seeds, he took to cultivating them ready to his hand, and when, in place of spending long hours in the hunt which at best could yield but a very limited supply of animal food, he learned to raise on his own account flocks and herds of oxen, sheep, goats, and pigs, and to breed birds of many varieties." One of the effects of the cultivation of food has been to make man more vegetarian than carnivorous, inasmuch as the land yields a more prolific supply of vegetable materials than of animal.

During the migratory period of agriculture, when patches of virgin soil were planted and abandoned for new ones as soon as the harvest was reaped, no great advance in civilization was made. Man still remained a hunter, combining hunting and fishing with desultory agriculture, and he still subsisted largely on the products of the uncultivated vegetable kingdom. In the later period—the period of stationary agriculture—when there was an abundance of animal and vegetable food materials, and when a large part of the total sum of human energy was liberated and made available for other purposes than the quest of food, a physiological division of labour was made possible, and social progress made headway.

The general effects of agriculture upon man's diet have been to accelerate the previous abandonment of raw vegetable food, and to increase the amount of starchy foods. The concentration of the diet, epoch by epoch, has become more and more marked, so that at the present time it forms the outstanding feature of the food of mankind. Another result of the development of agriculture and the cultivation of fruits, such as the date, the fig, the grape, and the banana, is the rapid increase in the quantity of sugar entering into man's diet.

The conclusions Dr. Campbell arrives at from his researches on the dietary of evolving man are—

1. The fact that man has evolved from the ape on a highly carnivorous diet disposes of the contention that man is essentially vegetarian by nature, and that meat and other animal foods are harmful.

2. The fact that up to the beginning of the agricultural period man's supply of sugar was scanty, whereas during it, and especially within recent times, it has been enormously increased, suggests that ill-health may often result from its excessive use. As a matter of experience in the dieting of patients, more good can be done by curtailing the starchy foods and sugar than by cutting down animal food, and this even in such diseases as gout and megrim.

3. So far as the general results affect the food of mankind, the ideal dietary is one that is simple in quality and moderate in quantity. It should contain a fair proportion, a quarter to one-third, of animal food. A certain amount of vegetable food should be uncooked in order to compel thorough mastication, and excess of sugar should be guarded against.

The general bearing of Dr. Campbell's work on the foodstuffs and diet of evolving man would be to show how very important a part has been played by the protein element. The food of existing precibiculturists is estimated as being composed of half animal and half vegetable material, so that the degree of nitrogenous interchange within the body should reach a high level.

Animal food, as contrasted with the types of vegetable foods available in those places where precibïculturists at present are to be found, is of far greater nutritive value. From experiments carried out in India, it will be shown that even with cultivated vegetable foodstuffs (barley, millets, etc.) the coefficient of protein absorption rarely reaches 60 per cent., while with animal food it is over 95 per cent. Even in the presimian period of man's evolution there would appear to have been a continuous struggle for the more concentrated forms of protein food, and particularly for the highly nitrogenous animal materials.

The Chemical Composition of Food Materials.

It is necessary in making a general survey of the food of mankind to take notice of the gross chemical composition of the different food materials. Analyses of practically every form of food have been made—at least for those entering into the dietaries in use in Europe and America. A very complete account of the work done in America will be found in Atwater and Bryant's "Chemical Composition of American Food Materials," Bulletin No. 28, U.S. Department of Agriculture. It will, therefore, only be necessary to refer to the chemical composition of some of the chief foodstuffs of European or American origin, whilst a full account of the composition of those peculiar to India and the tropics generally will be given, as the results hitherto obtained for these substances have not been widely circulated.

Accepting the ordinary classification of the organic chemical compounds or proximate principles of food materials as being conveniently grouped under the headings of protein, carbohydrate, and fats, it may be stated in very general terms, with regard to the protein element, that animal food shows from 20 to 25 per cent., legumes of different types almost an equal amount, cereals from 7 to 15 per cent., vegetables from 1 to 3 per cent., fruits about the same as vegetables, and nuts from 10 to 20 per cent. In the case of animal food the percentage of protein varies with the condition of the flesh and with the presence or absence of fat.

The first table on p. 32 gives the chemical composition of some of the chief European and American foods, the analyses being those of Atwater and Bryant.

In the second table are given the results of analyses of Indian foodstuffs; these analyses were made in India from samples of the food materials in use in the gaols of Bengal and the United

THE PROTEIN ELEMENT IN NUTRITION

Food Materials.	Water.	Protein.	Fat.	Carbohydrates.	Ash.	Fuel Value per Pound.
	Per Cent.	Per Cent.	Per Cent.	Per Cent.	Per Cent.	Calories
Beef, fresh : Brisket, medium fat	54·6	15·8	28·5	—	0·9	1,495
Ribs, lean	73·1	19·5	8·3	—	1·0	715
,, fat	52·0	16·5	31·1	—	0·8	1,620
Tongue	70·8	18·9	9·2	—	1·0	740
Lamb, fresh : Hindquarter	60·9	19·6	19·1	—	1·0	1,170
Mutton, fresh : Shoulder, medium fat	61·9	17·7	19·9	—	0·9	1,170
Pork, fresh : Ham, fresh	50·1	15·7	33·4	—	0·9	1,700
Bacon, smoked, average	20·2	10·5	64·8	—	5·1	2,930
Sausage, Pork, average	39·8	13·0	44·2	1·1	2·2	2,125
Chicken	74·8	21·5	2·5	—	1·1	505
Trout	77·8	19·2	2·1	—	1·2	445
Eggs	73·7	13·4	10·5	—	1·0	720
Butter	11·0	1·0	85·0	—	3·0	3,605
Cheese, Cheddar	27·4	27·7	36·8	4·1	4·0	2,145
Wheat flour, fine	13·8	7·9	1·4	76·4	0·5	1,625
entire wheat	11·4	13·8	1·9	71·9	1·0	1,675
Rice	12·3	8·0	0·3	79·0	0·4	1,630
Barley-meal	11·9	10·5	2·2	72·8	2·6	1,640
Oatmeal	7·3	16·1	7·2	67·5	1·9	1,860
Kafir corn	16·8	6·6	3·8	70·6	2·2	1,595
Rye flour	11·4	6·8	0·9	78·8	0·7	1,630
Carrots, fresh	88·2	1·1	0·4	9·3	1·0	210
Cauliflower	92·3	1·8	0·5	4·7	0·7	140
Peas, green	74·6	7·0	0·5	16·9	1·0	465
,, dried	9·5	24·6	1·0	62·0	2·9	1,655
Potatoes, raw	78·3	2·2	0·1	18·4	1·0	385
Bananas, yellow	75·3	1·3	0·6	22·0	0·8	460
Almonds	4·8	21·0	54·9	17·3	2·0	3,030
Walnuts	2·5	18·4	64·4	13·0	1·7	3,300

Food Materials.	Water.	Protein.	Carbohydrates.	Fat.	Ash.
	Per Cent.	Per Cent.	Per Cent.	Per Cent.	Per Cent.
Goat's flesh	—	24·06	—	2·50	1·10
Fish	—	17·80	—	5·04	—
Rice, Burma	11·13	6·95	77·25	0·96	1·34
,, country	11·05	6·62	81·07	0·50	1·04
Wheat flour	11·83	11·47	70·90	2·04	3·14
Maize (corn-meal)	11·50	9·52	68·90	4·44	3·75
Barley	—	8·92	76·10	1·90	—
Juar (a small millet)	—	7·67	67·26	2·77	—
Bajra (a large millet)	—	8·72	73·40	4·76	—
Mung dal (a legume)	10·87	23·62	53·45	2·69	3·57
Massur dal ,,	10·23	25·47	55·03	3·00	3·33
Gram dal ,,	10·07	19·91	54·22	4·34	4·69
Kalai dal ,,	10·87	22·58	58·02	1·10	3·61
Mattar dal ,,	10·96	22·01	53·97	1·96	3·60
Arhar dal ,,	10·08	21·70	54·06	2·50	5·50
Urid dal ,,	—	22·33	55·22	1·95	—

Provinces of Agra and Oudh. Only averages of the chemical composition are shown; full details will be found in the original papers.*

These results are the averages of a very large number of analyses carried out at different seasons of the year, during which the degree of moisture varies considerably.

Professor F. G. Benedict, of the Nutrition Laboratory of the Carnegie Institution of Washington, U.S.A., very kindly assisted in the examination of the Indian food materials. A tabular statement of the averages of his results for the moisture and the heat of combustion is appended :

Food Materials.	Water.	Heat of Combustion : Calories per Gramme.	Number of Determinations.
Wheat	10·58	3·951	14
Maize	9·97	4·094	4
Rice, Burma	10·27	3·820	4
,, country	10·75	3·805	4
Barley	13·47	3·752	4
Juar	11·13	3·913	2
Arhar dal	9·81	4·053	10
Gram dal	9·62	4·218	14
Kalai dal	10·19	4·034	4
Mattar dal	9·76	4·075	4
Massur dal	9·92	3·060	6
Mung dal	9·80	4·051	2
Urid dal	10·56	3·976	4

The moisture was determined by prolonged desiccation in a high vacuum, according to the method of Benedict and Manning. The heat of combustion was determined in a Kröker's calorimetric bomb by means of a new form of adiabatic calorimeter, designed by Benedict and Higgins. The hydrothermal equivalent to the calorimeter system was so taken that the heat of combustion of pure cane-sugar was 3,959 calories per gramme.

THE DIGESTIBILITY AND ABSORBABILITY OF FOODSTUFFS.

The food of mankind may now be considered from the standpoint of its real value—i.e., the amount of the food ingested that is actually taken up and made available for the requirements of the body. It is a mere truism to state that the gross chemical value of a food material may not necessarily be a measure of its real nutritive value, and that the real value depends on the degree of absorbability of its proximate principles; yet in many cases

* Scientific Memoirs, Government of India, Nos. 34, 37, and 48.

dietaries are framed on the results of chemical analyses alone, and little or no account taken of the absorption possible from the different foodstuffs. This may not be a matter of first importance when dealing with the high-class food materials made use of in Europe and America, or where an animal protein forms a substantial part of the nitrogenous intake, but it is of very real importance in the dieting of bodies of men with the vegetable foodstuffs of India and the tropics generally. Many of the dietaries framed for prisoners, famine camps, soldiers, etc., in India have been worked out from the gross chemical composition,

ABSORBABILITY OF DIFFERENT FOODS.

Food Materials.	Per Cent. Absorbed.			
	Dry Substance.	Protein.	Fat.	Carbohydrates.
Meat and fish	95	Practically all	79 to 92	—
Eggs	95	,,	96	—
Milk	91	88 to 100	93 to 98	?
Butter	—	—	98	—
Margarine	—	—	96	—
Fine wheat bread	95½	81 to 100	?	99
Decorticated whole wheat bread	88	69½	?	92½
Maize meal	93	89	?	97
Macaroni	95	81	?	97½
Rice	96	84	?	99
Peas	99	82½	?	96½
Beans	82	70	—	?
French beans	85	—	—	—
Potato puree (in small quantities)	—	80½	—	Practically all
Potatoes in general	80½	70	—	92½
Cabbage	85	81½	—	84½
Carrots	79	81½	—	82
Beetroots	—	72	?	82

so as to reach a certain standard, whilst no allowance was made for the fact that the absorption of the most important element, protein, from Indian vegetable food materials may be, and is in the majority of cases, very poor indeed. It is therefore of the greatest importance to know what the relative absorption is from the different types of foodstuffs in order that a clear conception may be formed of the real nutritive value of a food, and that in arranging dietaries they may be framed on their real worth, and not merely on their gross or apparent value.

Within comparatively recent years a great deal of work has been done in Europe and America with a view of ascertaining the coefficients of absorbability of the several constituents of the different foodstuffs. A great part of our knowledge on this subject is due to the admirable work done in the different nutrition laboratories in America in connection with the U.S. Department of Agriculture. Hutchison * summarizes the results in the table on p. 34, constructed from the figures of Rubner and Atwater.

From a large number of experiments on man, Langworthy † calculates that on an average the different groups into which foods may for convenience be divided have the following coefficients of digestibility :

COEFFICIENTS OF DIGESTIBILITY OF DIFFERENT GROUPS—PERCENTAGES.

	Protein.	Fat.	Carbohydrates.
Animal food	97	95	98
Cereals	85	90	98
Legumes, dried	78	90	97
Starches and sugars	—	—	98
Vegetables	83	90	95
Fruits	85	90	90
Vegetable foods	84	90	97
Total food	92	95	97

These figures show that the protein and fat of animal foods are much more completely absorbed than those of vegetables, with which there may be a loss in the fæces up to over 30 per cent. of the total protein consumed.

On the whole, however, it may be accepted that the foodstuffs in use in Europe and America show a high percentage of absorption for the several proximate principles. Animal protein is readily and completely digested, that of vegetables less completely. Fats are well digested, and carbohydrates show a high coefficient of absorbability, except when the amount of crude fibre or cellulose is large.

On a fruitarian diet the digestibility is not quite so good.

Jaffa gives the following results based on thirty digestion experiments with fruit dietaries :

Protein	..	..	..	..	75 per cent. absorbed.
Fat	..	..	..	..	86 ,, ,,
Sugar	..	..	..	..	95 ,, ,,
Fibre	..	..	..	..	79 ,, ,,
Calories	..	..	..	..	86 ,, ,,

---

* Hutchison, " Food and the Principles of Dietetics," 1911.
† Langworthy, Circular No. 46, U.S. Department of Agriculture.

CHAPTER III

TROPICAL FOOD MATERIALS AND THEIR DIGESTIBILITY

WHILE the digestibility of the different food materials entering into the composition of European and American dietaries has been very thoroughly worked out, up to quite recently no data were available for computing the true nutritive values of many of the vegetable foods of India and the tropics. A considerable amount of experimental work has been carried out during the last few years in determining the protein and carbohydrate absorption of the different classes of vegetable food materials peculiar to tropical countries.* It is necessary in a review of the digestibility of the foods of mankind to take into consideration the results arrived at, and contrast them with the values found for the absorption of protein from similar types of food materials made use of in other countries, as set forth in the previous chapter.

The common foodstuffs of India and the tropics generally are mostly derived from the vegetable kingdom. Some are peculiar to the tropics, being rarely seen in Europe; others are peculiarly tropical foods in that the quantities entering into the dietaries are very great, being out of all proportion to what would be consumed of the same food material by Europeans or Americans. These foodstuffs include rice, maize, wheat, barley, different millets, different legumes, vegetables, and fruits.

Rice, maize, wheat, and barley have been investigated, and the coefficients of absorption worked out, as shown in the above tables; but in dealing with the same food materials in India the local methods of preparing the grains for food have to be taken into consideration. These methods are rough and ready, and the resulting products are very dissimilar to the high-class preparations placed on the market in Europe. The ordinary method

* Scientific Memoirs, Government of India, Nos. 37 and 48.

of employing the cereals and legumes as food consists in separating the grain from the chaff and dirt, often very imperfectly; they are then washed, sun-dried, and ground between millstones into meal. The great mass of the population live, therefore, on a wholemeal dietary; in certain cases, however, some of the finer material is sifted out, and made use of in confectionery. In the larger towns and amongst the wealthier classes finer grades of flour prepared in properly equipped mills are made use of.

Rice forms the staple food of the great majority of the population of Lower Bengal, Eastern Bengal, and Assam, Burma, and the different parts of India where there is a sufficient supply of water for its cultivation. The rice in use is of two kinds—Burma rice and country rice. Burma, or Rangoon rice, the so-called "white" rice, is prepared direct from unhusked "paddy"—*i.e.*, as obtained from the rice-fields; it is milled by machinery, and the husk, pericarp, and surface layers of the seed are removed. The result is a clean white rice grain, deprived to some extent of its outer layers, and slightly of its protein and mineral constituents.

Indian, or country rice is prepared by soaking the "paddy" for from twenty-four to forty-eight hours in water; it is then transferred to lightly covered cylinders, in which it is steamed for from five to ten minutes; subsequently it is removed to open paved—usually sun-baked mud—courts, and dried by exposure to the sun. The sample obtained by this process is yellowish-brown in colour, and usually much contaminated with dirt. The outer layers of the grain, however, are not lost, so that, weight for weight, it should contain more protein and mineral matter than Burma rice.

Rice is the poorest of all cereals in protein; when cooked it swells up, and absorbs about three to three and a half times its weight of water. Very little of the protein is removed when it is boiled in a large quantity of water and the excess strained off. From analyses of the drained material there appears to be a loss of about 0·20 per cent. of the protein.

Being very deficient in the protein element, it will be obvious that, in order to obtain an adequate supply of this important material, a people whose diet consists almost wholly of rice must consume large quantities. This is found to be the case, and in all fixed dietaries where rice is the main constituent it is present in quantities up to and exceeding 26 ounces of the dried material. When it is borne in mind that rice swells up on being cooked to almost five times its dried bulk, it will be readily understood how voluminous a diet rice provides. It has been calculated that the gaol diet of Lower Bengal attains such a bulk on being cooked that an ordinary sized stomach would be required to be filled to the extreme limits of its capacity three times a day in order to accommodate the total amount. According to Hutchison, the total capacity of an ordinary sized European stomach is about 1,200 grammes, while the weight of a full gaol diet of rice exceeds 3,000 to 3,500 grammes.

Continental and American observers state that rice is absorbed with very great completeness in the intestine, while its progress through the stomach is slow. Thus Hutchison states that practically none of the starch is lost, but the waste of protein amounts to 19 per cent. Rubner and Atwater place the protein absorption at 84 per cent. Oshima,[*] in his digest of Japanese investigations, gives the average absorption of the protein of rice as 75·6 per cent., and of rice gruel as 56·1 per cent. These results, however, were obtained in the majority of cases when rice was eaten in comparatively small quantities. When the quantity of rice in the diet is large, the digestibility and protein absorption from it falls, and from the results of investigation on prisoners in India there is strong evidence that the protein absorption from rice, or from diets containing rice, varies largely with the actual volume or bulkiness of the diet.

In diet scales in Europe and America the question of bulk is not one of much importance ; the diets are very much concentrated, and are never sufficiently voluminous to cause distension of the stomach, while the contrary is commonly the condition met with when large quantities of rice are consumed. This question of bulk is a very important one from the standpoint of the absorption of protein. It was found in feeding experiments on prisoners in Bengal that when a diet was bulky out of all proportion to the nutriment it contained, the absorption of protein was greatly interfered with, and that by decreasing or increasing the quantity of rice in the diet, an increased or decreased absorption of protein takes place—*i.e.*, under certain conditions a decrease in the bulk of a diet will cause not only an

[*] Oshima, " A Digest of Japanese Investigations on the Nutrition of Man," U.S. Department of Agriculture, Bulletin No. 159.

increased percentage absorption of protein, but also an increase in the total amount of protein undergoing metabolism. The following results * of observations on this point will make the meaning clear:

In diets containing 30 ozs. of dry rice 6·55 grms. nitrogen were absorbed.
,,   ,,   26   ,,   ,,   7·55   ,,   ,,   ,,
,,   ,,   24   ,,   ,,   8·00   ,,   ,,   ,,
,,   ,,   23   ,,   ,,   8·09   ,,   ,,   ,,
,,   ,,   20   ,,   ,,   8·40   ,,   ,,   ,,
,,   ,,   19   ,,   ,,   8·47   ,,   ,,   ,,

The explanation of a decrease in the amount of nitrogenous interchange, as the bulk of a diet increases beyond a certain point, is in all probability due to the difficulty experienced by the digestive juices in penetrating the mass, and to dilatation and weakening of the walls of the stomach, inducing a loss of power in the passing on of its contents. Perhaps even more important is the fact that the large mass on reaching the intestines sets up increased peristalsis, so that the contents are hurried on into the large intestine, where protein absorption is at a minimum. The large watery or semi-solid stools passed by prisoners fed on large quantities of rice would lend support to this view.

It will be obvious from what has been said that where bulk interferes with the protein absorption from a diet no fixed co-efficient for the absorption of the protein of its constituents can be possible. For each separate quantity of rice above a certain amount a different percentage of its contained protein will be absorbed. This was found to be the explanation of the results obtained for the variations in the percentage of protein absorption met with in the bulky diets of prisoners in the gaols of Bengal, and in all probability it would assist in explaining the varying coefficients of the digestibility of rice given by other observers. In Oshima's list the protein absorption of rice ranged in different experiments from 46·5 to 86·4 per cent. Aron confirms the results obtained for the protein absorption of rice. His figures vary from 53 to 68 per cent.†

The decrease in the coefficient of protein absorption with diets containing large amounts of rice may be so great that the total nitrogenous absorption may fall to little more than 50 per cent. of the protein presented in the diet. Thus, on an average, over a large number of experiments on batches of prisoners under

* Scientific Memoirs, Government of India, No. 37, Chart I.
† Aron and Hocson, " Rice as Food," *Philippine Journal of Science*, 1911.

observation for varying periods of from five to ten days, the percentage of protein absorption from diets containing about 26 ounces of rice—the other constituents being contant—works out to be 54·28 per cent. As the quantity of rice was reduced—the other constituents of the dietary remaining constant—the percentage absorption of protein gradually rose,* thus—

Diet containing 32 ozs. of rice showed 6·55 grms. N. absorption, or 45·76 %
,,   ,,   26   ,,   ,,   7·85   ,,   ,,   ,,   53·66 ,,
,,   ,,   24   ,,   ,,   8·00   ,,   ,,   ,,   55·39 ,,
,,   ,,   23   ,,   ,,   8·09   ,,   ,,   ,,   59·69 ,,
,,   ,,   20   ,,   ,,   8·40   ,,   ,,   ,,   64·03 ,,
,,   ,,   19   ,,   ,,   8·47   ,,   ,,   ,,   68·33 ,,

There can be little doubt that with diets in which rice forms only a small element, in an otherwise non-bulky diet, the percentage absorption of the protein of rice would be comparatively high, probably up to the figure given by Atwater—viz., 84 per cent.

But not only does the great bulk of rice when cooked cause interference with the protein absorption from the rice itself, but it also causes the nitrogenous element of the other constituents of the diet to be less readily absorbed. The same explanation given for the relatively poor absorption of the protein of rice in a bulky diet would hold for any other constituents—the whole mass in the stomach having little opportunity of being thoroughly mixed with gastric juice, and, after leaving the stomach, being hurried on past the parts where absorption is best carried out into the large intestine, where absorption is at a minimum. As an illustration of the influence of the volume of diets on the absorption of the protein of its component, the results† obtained in feeding a batch of prisoners for a week on each of the following diets may be cited :

Constants.	Varying Amounts of Rice.	Absorption of Nitrogen per Man Daily.	Per Cent. of Nitrogen Absorbed.	Diet.
Wheat .. 10 ozs. Arhar dal.. 6 ,, Vegetables 6 ,,	16 ozs. 14 ,, 12 ,, 10 ,, 8 ,,	9·71 grms. 10·10 ,, 10·49 ,, 9·86 ,, 9·78 ,,	56·96 61·52 66·45 64·95 67·23	I. II. III. IV. V.

From these results it is evident that a decrease in the amount of rice from 16 to 12 ounces causes both a relative and actual

* Scientific Memoirs, Government of India, No. 37, p. 61.
† *Ibid.*, No. 37, Chart VIII., p. 132.

increase in the amount of protein undergoing metabolism ; also, when Diets III. and IV., or IV. and V., are contrasted, the fact that there must be an accompanying increased absorption from the "constants" of the diets will be clear. Thus—

Diet III. N. of constants+ 3·74 grms. N. from rice, 10·49 grms. absorbed,
,,   IV.   ,,   ,,   + 3·12   ,,   ,,   9·86   ,,   ,,

which would mean, if the increase of nitrogen absorption all came from the extra rice in Diet III., that 0·62 gramme gave an absorption of 0·63 gramme. This is impossible, and the explanation simply is that there is a greater amount of protein absorbed from the "constants" and from the rice when the bulk of the diet is decreased. A similar comparison of Diets IV. and V. exemplified this also.

If the Diets I., II., and III. be examined, it will be found that where the amount of rice is beyond the optimum, in this combination, 12 ounces, the reverse conditions obtain. As the rice increases in quantity, and the bulk of the diet becomes greater, a lower and lower percentage of protein absorption takes place from both "constants," and from the varying quantities of rice.

These results serve to illustrate the impossibility of obtaining any fixed figures for the coefficients of the protein absorption of rice, or other foodstuffs of a bulky nature, when the quantities of the food materials entering into the composition of the dietaries are large. Under such conditions they also show that when a bulky food, such as rice, is combined with other materials, not in themselves bulky, the degree of protein absorption from both the rice and the other foodstuffs varies inversely with the total volume of the diet.

It is quite different when food materials of a more concentrated nature are experimented with, and when bulk does not cause any interference with protein absorption.

In connection with the poor protein absorption obtained from vegetable dietaries, Hutchison, quoting Hofman, states that in a number of prison diets of an exclusively vegetable nature. it was found that on an average from 25 to 47 per cent. of the protein escaped absorption—results that are very much the same as those obtained in investigating the nutritive values of the vegetable gaol dietaries of Bengal.

Hutchison has collected the results of a number of experiments on the absorption of protein with vegetable foods, contrasting them with that of the protein of meat :*

RELATIVE ABSORPTION OF PROTEIN IN VARIOUS FOODS.

Diet.	Protein not Absorbed.
Meat	2·3 per cent.
Lentil flour	10·5 ,,
Dried peas	17·0 ,,
Beans } Flour }	30·3 ,,
Potatoes	32·0
Carrots and fat	39·0 ,,
Lentils (simply soaked and boiled till soft)..	40·0 ,,

In dealing with the other cereals utilized in India as food, no great difficulty was experienced in obtaining fairly constant figures for the coefficients of protein absorption, as, except in the case of rice, the question of bulk is not a serious one. On the other hand, the ordinary foodstuffs are very much mixed with one another, and often greatly contaminated with foreign grains, so that pure samples are difficult to obtain. The effect of this is that variations in the figures representing the nitrogen absorption are met with, unless the same sample is used throughout the experiments.

Wheat is by far the most important of the cereals used as food in India. It is prepared for consumption by grinding with small hand-driven grinding-stones, the whole grain being so treated. The bran is partially got rid of by sifting, but the germ remains, the meal, or *ata*, consisting of the products of the germ and endosperm. The wheat is always freshly ground every few days, so that there is no difficulty over the oil in the germ turning rancid. The *ata*, or meal, which contains the products of the whole wheat grain except the coarser elements of the bran, is baked with water and salt into unleavened bread, usually in the form of flat cakes, called *chapatti* or *roti*. A mixture of wheaten and barley flour is employed in some districts for making the *chapatti*, but in the majority of cases the wheat crop is grown contaminated, particularly with barley, so that pure samples of wheat are difficult to obtain. In the poorer samples of wheat all manner of grains are to be found—barley, gram, maize, linseed, etc. ; some of these will tend to raise the protein content of the sample, while decreasing its coefficient of protein absorption, while some will tend to lower the protein content and relative absorption at the same time. In the case of fairly clean samples, however, the contamination is mainly due to barley, so that the tendency is for a fall in the protein content to be accompanied by a fall in the percentage of nitrogen absorbed. Thus, in contrasting some of the results obtained for the protein content and protein absorption of different samples of wheat, it was found that—

1 oz. first class Benares wheat contains 0·5354 grm. N., of which 80·5 per cent. is absorbed.
1 oz. first class Agra wheat contains 0·4896 grm. N., of which 72·3 per cent. is absorbed.
1 oz. ordinary Naini wheat contains 0·4710 grm. N., of which 68·8 per cent. is absorbed.
1 oz. ordinary Benares and Lucknow wheat contains 0·4630 grm. N., of which 69·2 per cent. is absorbed.

It would appear from these findings that a relationship exists between the protein content of a sample and the percentage of protein absorption from that sample. While this may be true for samples that are fairly clean and pure, or in which the only or chief foreign element is barley, it does not hold good for all classes of wheat, nor when the containing factors are of various kinds. Thus—

1 oz. ordinary Agra wheat contains 0·4536 grm. N., of which 63·3 per cent. is absorbed.
1 oz. ordinary Lucknow wheat contains 0·4360 grm. N., of which 67·5 per cent. is absorbed.
1 oz. ordinary Lucknow wheat contains 0·4415 grm. N., of which 71·4 per cent. is absorbed.

So that, although the ordinary sample of Agra wheat contains a higher percentage of nitrogen than either of the Lucknow samples, yet it is accompanied by a percentage of protein absorption considerably lower than was found in the case of the latter.

It may be accepted, therefore, that in India, while really good, clean wheat shows a protein absorption of over 80 per cent., thus comparing very favourably with the results given by European and American authorities, the ordinary contaminated material available to the great mass of the population is not nearly so well absorbed, the coefficient of protein digestibility varying in different samples from 62·8 to 72·3 per cent.

Experimenting in India on batches of from five to ten prisoners kept under observation for periods varying from five to ten days, it was found that the absorption of the protein of good wheat varied within narrow limits.

The following results were obtained :

Observations* Nos. 21 and 22	..	80·8 per cent. of nitrogen absorbed.
,, ,, 23 ,, 24	..	80·4 ,, ,, ,,
Observation No. 28	.. ..	79·3 ,, ...
,, ,, 30	.. ..	81·0 ,, ,, ,,
,, ,, 32	.. ..	80·8 ,, ,, ,,

The average absorption of the protein of this wheat is, therefore, practically 80·5 per cent. These results were all obtained from the same sample of wheat. The wheat was specially selected as being clean and pure for the purpose of the experiment. It was ground in hand-driven stone-mills, and contained all the elements of the grain, except the coarser parts of the bran, which were rejected on sifting. An absorption of over 80 per cent. of the protein of all the elements of the wheat grain, including the germ, therefore, may be expected when the sample of wheat is pure and in good condition.

But no such favourable results are obtained when the sample of wheat is contaminated and dirty. From the results of observations carried out on a large scale in four large gaols of the United Provinces, the protein absorption, shown by the different wheats experimented with, was found to vary with the condition of the sample. Taking an average of the results given by feeding experiments with ordinary wheat as supplied, the protein absorption works out as follows :

Observations† Nos. 25 and 26..	..	69·3 per cent. absorbed.
Observation No. 31	.. ..	68·3 ,, ,,
Observations Nos. 51, 52, and 53	..	62·8 ,, ,,
,, ,, 57, 58, and 59	..	69·7 ,, ,,
,, ,, 60 and 61	..	67·9 ,, ,,
,, ,, 63, 64, and 65	..	71·4 ,, ,,
Observation No. 72	.. ..	67·5 ,, ,,
,, ,, 84	.. ..	72·3 ,, ,,
Observations Nos. 77, 78, and 79	..	63·1 ,, ,,

That is, taking the protein absorption, where different samples of common wheat were experimented with, the average quantity made use of in the body works out at 68 per cent.

For the very large proportion of the wheat consumed by the masses in India, this percentage of protein absorption is all that could be counted on. It is not altogether a matter of adulteration by the seller, as not infrequently a mixture of cereals, such as wheat and barley, is cultivated as such. The majority of the population live by agriculture, and grow their own foodstuffs, which are ground and prepared by the women-folk in their own homes. Except in the large towns, there is practically no buying of ground wheat or other foodstuffs.

* Scientific Memoirs, Government of India, No. 48. † *Loc. cit.*

So far as information is available, there are practically no results of experimental work recorded where the whole grain of the wheat is utilized. Goodfellow, in investigating the nutritive value of Hovis bread—in which the germ is partially cooked with superheated steam, ground to meal, and added to the ordinary flour—found the percentage of protein absorption very little lower than with ordinary white bread. It is important, therefore, to remember that when dealing with a good quality of wheat, the protein absorption from the flour containing all the elements of the grain, except the coarser parts of the bran, is slightly over 80 per cent., and, further, that the protein content of the wheat has not been impoverished by the exclusion of the highly nitrogenous germ. In the particular sample of wheat referred to, and with which the above result was obtained, the amount of protein present was 12 per cent.

It is necessary now to examine the effect of the modern methods of milling wheat on the protein content of the products obtained.

Hutchison gives the composition of the different parts of a wheat grain as follows :

	Bran: 13·5 per Cent.	Endosperm: 85 per Cent.	Germ: 1·5 per Cent.	Whole Grain: 100 per Cent.
Water	12·5	13·0	12·5	14·5
Nitrogenous matter	16·4	10·5	35·7	11·0
Fat	3·5	0·8	13·1	1·2
Starch and sugar	43·6	74·3	31·2	69·0
Cellulose	18·0	0·7	1·8	2·6
Mineral water	6·0	0·7	5·7	1·7

In the old method of stone-grinding—the method still in use in India—the bran was removed, but not the germ; whereas in the modern steel-roller milling both bran and germ are excluded. After being ground, the products are separated into different portions by sifting, and the portion that constitutes flour is derived entirely from the endosperm, and forms from 70 to 73 per cent. of the whole grain. This flour is further separated into a portion derived from the central part of the endosperm, which is poor in protein and rich in starch. This is termed " patents "; the remaining portion is the ordinary household or baker's flour. Neglecting further refinements in the division of the products, the effect of modern methods of milling is to lessen very considerably the protein and mineral constituents of the flour. Thus Hutchison compares the different preparations as follows :

	Wheat-meal.	Medium Flour: Households or Baker's.	Finest Flour: Patents.
Nitrogenous matter	14·2 per cent.	10·7 per cent.	7·9 per cent.
Fat	1·9 ,,	1·1 ,,	1·4 ,,
Carbohydrates	70·6 ,,	75·4 ,,	76·4 ,,
Ash	1·2 ,,	0·5 ,,	0·5 ,,

There are factors, however, which tend to counteract this loss of protein : thus the very whitest flour—" patents "—is generally used for fancy bread and pastry ; the ordinary flour is a blend of different wheats selected as the most suitable for bread-making. The suitability depends on " strength," which in its turn depends on the percentage of gluten ; so that the protein element can never fall very low, otherwise the flour would not make bread at all. Again, according to some authorities, the protein content of different wheats varies enormously,[*] so that the exclusion of the germ would make little difference in comparison with the difference between flour made from different varieties of wheat.

Quite recently an outcry has arisen against the composition of the fine white bread at present placed on the market, and a demand made for the improvement of the finer high-grade flours, particularly in their nitrogenous and mineral constituents. As already pointed out, with the present processes of milling about 70 per cent. of the wheat grain is utilized as flour. In the improvement advocated a standard bread was demanded, the proposal being that not less than 80 per cent. of the grain should be made use of in the manufacture of flour, and that this should contain the germ of the wheat grain and the semolina.

The advantages claimed for "standard" bread are—It contains a higher proportion of iron and phosphorus in a state of combination capable of absorption ; other mineral constituents are also higher, which is a point of great importance in the formation of bone and teeth. It has not been impoverished by the loss of the germ and part of the outer layers, so that it contains a higher percentage of protein and fat than white bread. The presence of a small portion of the bran acts as a mechanical stimulus to the digestive tract, thus lessening the tendency to constipa-

[*] No great differences in the protein content of wheat were met with in the analyses of various samples made in India. The results obtained were fairly uniform, so long as clean, pure wheat was examined.

tion. Certain other advantages of minor importance are also claimed.

There is very little doubt of the truth of these claims for the superiority of "standard" flour when contrasted with white flour manufactured from the same class of wheat, and with the same care in mixing wheats from different sources, as millers state is the custom at present in order to obtain a strong flour, it is difficult to see how this "standard" flour would not maintain its superiority. In other words, under the same conditions of manufacturing, "standard" flour should show the above-mentioned points of superiority when contrasted with the ordinary white flour milled from the same source. A "standard" flour obtained from a low-class wheat might in all probability be inferior in nutritive value to ordinary white flour milled from a high-class wheat, and it has been asserted that the "standard" flour allows millers to make use of inferior and injurious wheats, which could not be utilized in the preparation of good white flour. The report, however, of the medical department of the Local Government Board * on the bleaching of flours would show that millers can and do make use of inferior wheats in the production of white flour; the dark or injured parts can be bleached to represent the finest flour of high-grade wheat. The report states that bleaching with nitrogen peroxide, carefully carried out, in itself produces no appreciable effect upon the baking qualities of flour, but it is capable of improving the colour, and therefore the commercial value, of the lower grades of flour, enabling a low-priced article to simulate the appearance of a high-priced one. The report† goes on to show that the alterations in, and the additions to, flour which result from a high degree of bleaching by nitrogen peroxide cannot be regarded as free from risk to the consumer. It is demonstrated that there is a certain amount of nitrite-reacting material present in bleached flour, one of the effects of which is to cause interference with digestion. Thus, Halliburton found that traces of nitrites exert a distinct inhibitory effect on both proteolytic and amylolytic enzymes, 1 part of sodium nitrite in 8,000 inhibiting peptic digestion entirely, while 1 part in 32,000 decreased the power of the enzymes to one-seventh of its normal activity; similar results were obtained in the case of the salivary digestion of starch. Hale has found that sodium

* Reports to the Local Government Board on Public Health and Medical Subjects, Nos. 46 and 47.
† "The Purity of Flour and Bread," *British Medical Journal*, vol. i., 1911.

nitrite in a dilution of 1 part in 5,000 to 200,000 has a distinct inhibiting action on gastric digestion. Harden also showed a distinct, though small, inhibition in the peptic digestion of samples of bleached flour as compared with unbleached.

Another method by which the millers are able to make use of inferior wheats in the production of the finest white flours is by the addition of "improvers." These were found to consist essentially of phosphoric acid, or acid phosphates of calcium, magnesium, potassium, phosphorus trichloride, and pentachloride, oxides and sulphides of phosphorus, acids such as iodic, hydrofluoric, formic, acetic, propionic, etc., alcohol, aldehyde, and ketones. The claim for these is that more bread can be obtained per sack of flour by their use, which simply means that more water can be supplied to the consumer at the price of bread. The protein content of flour is an important matter from the standpoint of nutrition, especially where bread enters largely into the diet. Flour from weak wheats, which are generally poor in gluten, contain less protein than flour from strong wheats, which are rich in gluten. But by the use of "improvers" flour from weak wheat is made to simulate flour from a stronger wheat, although much inferior to it in protein.

The indiscriminate addition of such substances as strong hydrofluoric acid, phosphorus pentachloride, oxides and sulphides of phosphorus, etc., to flour is most dangerous. It does not appear desirable that such an indispensable foodstuff as flour, the purity and wholesomeness of which are of first importance to the community, should be manipulated and treated with foreign substances whose utility from the point of view of the consumer is more than questionable.*

The general conclusion to be drawn from the result of these investigations is that millers, in the desire to produce fine flour of dazzling whiteness at as great a profit to themselves as possible, have considerably impoverished the flour in its protein content, fat, and mineral constituents; that, in order to be able to make use of inferior wheats, or increase the commercial value of the flour, they have introduced a method of bleaching with nitrogen peroxide gas, and a system of improving the "strength" of low-grade flours by the addition of foreign chemical substances. Neither the effects of the bleaching processes nor the addition of "improvers" in any way increases the dietetic value of the

* *Lancet,* Local Government Reports, vol. i., 1911.

bread to the consumer, while evidence is not wanting that these innovations are distinctly harmful, and may even be dangerous.

It may be concluded, therefore, that while a " standard " flour, containing 80 per cent. of the whole grain, and including the germ and semolina, permits of millers making use of inferior grades of wheat for its production—a deception that is already practised, and capable of considerable extension in the manufacture of ordinary white flour—at least, it gives no incentive to the gross adulteration of flour with harmful chemical substances, which, from the Government report above referred to, would appear to be only too common.

It is quite evident that in the evolution of the modern processes of milling, so far as the nutritive value of flour is concerned, a false standard has been set up—viz., one based on the colour, lightness, and texture of the products. In order to approach as nearly as possible to this standard, and at the same time produce a flour that will give the largest yield of the most attractive bread from a given quality of wheat, millers have not scrupled to reduce materially the important nutritive constituents of the flour, and to enhance its commercial value by methods that are distinctly deceptive, and in their effects not without danger to the public. If the only true criterion of a high-class flour—viz., the real nutritive value of the bread obtained therefrom—were adjudged the standard by which flours would be graded, there is very little doubt that millers would soon find it was to their own interests to place flour on the market that would meet all requirements, and all danger from inferior wheats and from adulteration with noxious compounds would be at an end.

From the results of feeding experiments carried out on a large scale in India with wholemeal obtained by grinding a good-class wheat, it has already been shown that 80 per cent. of the protein will be absorbed. This wholemeal has not been deprived of any of its nutritive material, and probably contains a slightly larger amount of the bran and outer layers than would be the case in " standard " bread. An equally high percentage of protein absorption should be possible from " standard " flour milled from a good class of wheat.

In another connection it will be necessary to consider the effects on the system of the retention of as much of the wheat grain as possible in flour; at present the relative degrees of absorption shown by different grades of flour require examination.

From an average of a considerable number of experiments by Rubner, Atwater, Zuntz and Magnus-Levy, Goodfellow, and others, Hutchison works out the loss of the nutritive constituents of wholemeal and white bread, when it formed the main part of the diet, as follows :

Constituents.	White Bread.	Wholemeal Bread.
Total solids	4·5 per cent.	14·0 per cent.
Protein	20·0 ,,	20 to 30 per cent.
Ash	25·0 ,,	51·0 ,,
Carbohydrates	3·0 ,,	6·0 ,,

There seems to be a considerable degree of confusion with regard to the terms used in the description of breads. Thus brown and wholemeal are used synonymously to apply to bread prepared from flour containing part of the bran, but not the germ; whereas real wholemeal flour should contain the germ in addition. There is a good deal of evidence that a large proportion of the brown or wholemeal bread placed on the market is prepared from low-grade flour, to which has been added a certain amount of bran. As might be expected, the absorption of the nutritive constituents of such bread must necessarily be poor.

The most recent work on the absorption of the constituents of different flours is that carried out by Professor Snyder in Minneapolis for the U.S. Department of Agriculture. Young healthy men were fed on bread prepared from three flours :

1. Graham, made by grinding the whole wheat.
2. Entire wheat, corresponding approximately to "standard" bread—includes the germ and semolina.
3. Patent, ordinary white flour of best quality.

The proportions assimilated were ascertained by analyses of the food taken, and of the total excreta over a period of time in the usual way. The results obtained were—

Different Flours.	Protein Absorbed.	Carbohydrate Absorbed.
Graham flour	74·9 per cent.	89·2 per cent.
Entire ,,	82·0 ,,	93·5 ,,
Patent ,,	88·6 ,,	97·7 ,,

These figures may be accepted as being as accurate as it is possible to obtain with a material that varies in its chemical composition so much as wheat. It will be evident that the old-fashioned household bread, "standard" bread, and the bread prepared from *ata* in India—all of which contain the germ and semolina—approximate closely to one another in their proximate principles, and show practically identical percentages of absorption and assimilation. The following table gives the results arrived at :

Different Flours.	Protein Present.	Protein Absorbed.	Carbohydrates Present.	Carbohydrates Absorbed.
	Per Cent.	Per Cent.	Per Cent.	Per Cent.
"Patent" flour	7·9	88·6	76·4	97·7
"Standard" flour		82·0	70·0	93·5
India *ata*	11·5 to 14·2	80·5	70·9	96·5
Old-fashioned household flour		80·0	70·0	95·0

It may therefore be concluded that while the protein element of the fine white flours is slightly better absorbed than in the case of real wholemeal or "standard" flour, the decided inferiority it shows in the amount of protein presented lessens its dietetic value very considerably, and, in the case of those with whom bread constitutes the main source of nutriment, entails a much lower level of nitrogenous interchange than would be attained on a similar quantity of flour containing the highly albuminous germ and semolina. Thus, for instance, a person living on 1,000 grammes of "patent" flour, and another on 1,000 grammes of "standard" flour, *ata*, or the old household flour, the first, with "patent" flour, would attain a level of nitrogenous metabolism equal to 79 multiplied by 0·88, or about 69·6 grammes of protein per day. The second, taking the average protein content at 12·5 per cent., and the coefficient of absorption at 81 per cent., would metabolize 101·25 grammes of protein per day. So that, from the standpoint of protein interchange within the body, the modern impoverishing methods of milling may affect very seriously the dietetic value of bread, and thus lower the stamina of those largely dependent on it for their nutrition. Leaving out of consideration the harmful effects of bleaching and the addition of so-called "improvers," there can be little doubt of the superiority of real wholemeal bread to ordinary white bread in protein content, and in the level of protein metabolism possible of attainment. But in addition to this there is another factor to be taken into consideration—viz., the relative values of white and wheat-meal breads on the growth and development of the body; this is probably associated with other constituents of the wheat grain besides protein. A large number of experiments have now been carried out with the view of contrasting the values of white bread, " standard " bread, and wholemeal bread in nutrition and growth. Flack and Hill have shown that white bread is very inferior from this standpoint. It is not necessary to enter into details; all that need be said at present is that the superiority of wheat as a foodstuff appears to be due partly to gluten and partly to an organic base. A similar base can be extracted from the pericarp of rice or outer layers of the rice grain by acid alcohol. It is not a phosphorized compound. The absence of this from white rice apparently is the cause of beri-beri.* There is a considerable amount of evidence that white flour is depleted to a very large extent of this important organic base, whilst, on the other hand, it is present in sufficient quantity in "standard" and real wholemeal flour to meet the requirements of the body.

Another typical Indian food material is maize or Indian corn. It is prepared for use in different ways. Usually the grain is ground to meal in exactly the same way as wheat. Sometimes the individual grains are separated from the cob and roasted, when they swell up and burst; in this form it is similar to the American popcorn. Often the cob, with adherent grains, is roasted; the maize is then eaten with butter and salt. Maize is extensively employed as a food material by the people of Behar, United Provinces, and other parts of India suitable for its cultivation; strangely enough, it is not used to any great extent in the feeding of prisoners.

In India the average protein content of maize was found to be 9·55 per cent., fully 2·5 per cent. less than wheat contains. Its fat is higher than any of the other Indian cereals, being almost twice as high as in wheat. As already pointed out, zein is the typical protein of maize, and it differs in its properties from the gluten of wheat or the proteins of other cereals. Owing to the absence of gluten corn-meal, cannot be baked into porous leaves like wheaten-meal. The bread is usually, therefore, of the unleavened type, and is of a granular appearance. The germ and husk are removed in the modern methods of milling, and the

---

* Casimir Funk has recently isolated this body, which he terms "the beri-beri vitamine," from the polishings of rice. He has determined its chemical nature, and demonstrated its wonderful effects on the polyneuritis set up in fowls by a diet of rice deprived of this substance (*Journal of Physiology*, December, 1911).

remaining endosperm is ground alone and purified by means of air currents. About 30 to 35 per cent. of the entire weight of the grain is rejected as offal, which consists of the hull, germ, floury particles, and some of the flinty portions of the corn. The effect of these losses is to lessen the protein, fat, and mineral constituents, and raise the carbohydrates. Thus—

Different Forms of Maize.	Protein.	Fat.	Carbohydrates.	Mineral Matters.
	Per Cent.	Per Cent.	Per Cent.	Per Cent.
Indian-corn	9·7	5·4	68·9	1·5
Corn meal	8·5	4·6	72·8	1·3
,, (fine)	6·8	1·3	78·0	0·6

This method of milling has almost entirely replaced the old-fashioned crushing of the corn between grooved mill-stones to the desired fineness—the coarse particles of the skin and bran only being rejected. In India the old method is the only one in use, so that it is corn-meal or wholemeal that is employed as food material.

Maize-meal, either baked or in the form of porridge, is very well digested and absorbed by the intestinal tract. In a large number of experiments* on prisoners in Bengal where maize was given along with rice, it was found that the protein element was as well absorbed as that of wheat, when the two foodstuffs were given under the same conditions.

Rubner † places the absorption of the protein of maize at 81·8 per cent., and its dry matter at 82 per cent. Later work on the digestibility of foods prepared from corn-meal in America would show that the protein constituent is slightly less thoroughly digested than that of wheat; but the difference is too slight to be of much practical importance. Thus, Harcourt states that 74 per cent. of the protein and 99 per cent. of the carbohydrates of corn-meal porridge are absorbed, and experiments at the Marine Experiment Station gave similar figures. With the finer cornmeals from which the germ, hull, and other coarser particles have been removed, the absorption of protein ranges from 77 to 86 per cent. The carbohydrates are almost completely utilized by the body. Of the different cereals experimented with in India, maize is decidedly superior to all with the exception of wheat; it is, therefore, difficult to understand why greater

* Scientific Memoirs, Government of India, No. 37, p. 158.
† Rubner. Zeit. f. Biolog., 1879, xv.

advantage of it is not taken in the feeding of prisoners. In America and Italy it forms the principal food for the majority of the rural population. In 1900 one-third of the land under cultivation in the United States was devoted to the maize crop, and it forms 5 per cent. of the cropped area of the United Provinces of India.

Maize has been popularly regarded as indigestible; as a good winter food, but too "heating" for summer use. How these ideas originated it is difficult to say; they obtain no support either from experimental work nor from the almost universal use made of it in the Southern United States, Mexico, and Mediterranean regions. Woods * sums up a discussion on its merits by saying—

"That it is wholesome and well suited to its numerous uses as a food material is abundantly proved by its long-continued use under a great variety of circumstances and conditions, and the high opinion in which it has always been held. Scientific investigations have abundantly justified the popular conclusions on the subject."

Another great advantage of maize is its cheapness. Of all the cereals it provides a greater return in protein, fat, carbohydrates, and energy for the same outlay.

It seems a pity that greater use is not made of such an excellent and cheap food by the poorer classes in Europe and in the feeding of prisoners in India. The Chinese employ maize very extensively, and on it are able to endure great fatigue, whilst their general physique and stamina reach a high level.

Of the other cereals utilized as foodstuffs in India that have been investigated—barley, juar, bajra, and marna—little need be said. They are all much inferior to wheat or maize in their gross chemical constituents, and in the amount of assimilable material they contain.

Barley (*Hordeum vulgare*) in India is usually grown mixed with pulses, sometimes with wheat. Both alone and in admixtures it is generally considered difficult of digestion. It is chiefly used in the form of powder or flour of the parched grain.

The analyses of Indian barley-meal† showed—

Protein	8·92 per cent.
Carbohydrates	76·10 ,,
Fat	1·90 ,,

---

* Woods, "Food Value of Corn Products," Bulletin No. 298, U.S. Department of Agriculture.

† Scientific Memoirs, Government of India, No. 48.

From an average of the results obtained in feeding experiments on batches of Indian prisoners, the absorption of the nitrogenous and carbohydrate constituents worked out to be—protein, 57·6 per cent.; carbohydrates, 96·0 per cent.* In his digestion experiments on the Japanese, Oshima† found practically identical figures—viz., protein, 59·8 per cent.; carbohydrates, 96·7 per cent., absorbed.

In dietaries where barley is substituted for part of the wheat, the average percentage of protein absorption falls, the extent of the fall depending on the degree of substitution. This takes place on an extensive scale all over India, as the wheat is grown largely mixed with barley, so that on being ground to meal there is obtained a mixture of wheat and barley. The protein absorption from this mixture usually averages between 65 and 70 per cent.

Juar (*Andropogon Sorghum* or *Sorghum vulgare*) is one of the high-growing millets. It is seldom grown alone, usually with some of the creeping pulses. Juar is one of the most important of the rainy-season crops of India, forming with rice and wheat the chief staple foods of the country. It is ground to meal, and from it are prepared unleavened bread, porridge, and other preparations. Its chemical composition was found to be—

Protein	7·67 per cent.
Carbohydrates	67·26 ,,
Fat	2·77 ,,

Like barley, it shows very defective protein absorption, the average over a large number of feeding experiments being—protein, 53 per cent.; carbohydrates, 97·8 per cent., absorbed.

Bajra (*Pennisetum typhoideum*) is another large millet. As an article of food it is much esteemed in some parts of India. The seeds are ground to meal and baked into cakes, or it is prepared as porridge. Boiled with milk, it is said to form a light and pleasant meal for invalids. The chemical composition of this food was found to be—

Protein	8·72 per cent.
Carbohydrates	73·40 ,,
Fat	1·90 ,,

Over a large number of observations, the average protein absorption worked out inferior to that of all other cereals, being only 49·4 per cent.

* Scientific Memoirs, Government of India, No. 48.
† Oshima, U.S. Department of Agriculture, Bulletin No. 159.

These three foodstuffs, barley, juar, and bajra, are very inferior when used alone or as the main constituent of a diet, as they exhibit so poor an absolute and relative absorption of the protein element. Thus, to take as examples* three of the ordinary diets arranged for prisoners in India, the following are the results :

Bajra	24 ozs.
Dals	6 ,,
Vegetables	6 ,,

Intake of nitrogen, 15·9798 grms.

Of this 9·5291 grammes of nitrogen were absorbed, or 59·6 per cent. of the total nitrogen offered in the diet.

Juar	22 ozs.
Dals	8 ,,
Vegetables	6 ,,

Intake of nitrogen, 16·2748 grms.

Of this 8·9992 grammes of nitrogen were absorbed, or 55·3 per cent. of the total nitrogen offered in the diet.

Barley	22 ozs.
Wheat	6 ,,
Dals	2 ,,
Vegetables	6 ,,

Intake of nitrogen, 14·3793 grms.

Of this 9·2264 grammes of nitrogen were absorbed, or 64·1 per cent. of the total nitrogen offered in the diet.

These results should be contrasted with the level of nitrogenous metabolism attained on a diet where a good class of wheat forms the principal cereal† :

Wheat	23 ozs.
Dals	4 ,,
Vegetables	6 ,,

Intake of nitrogen, 16·714 grms.

Of this 13·651 grammes of nitrogen were absorbed, or 81·6 per cent. of the nitrogen offered in the diet.

It will be evident from these results that there is a very large nitrogenous residue left over in the intestinal canal when food materials with a low coefficient of protein absorption, such as barley, juar, or bajra, form the main part of the diet. This residue provides a splendid culture medium for the growth of putrefactive micro-organisms, and is therefore likely to predispose to diarrhœa, dysentery, and other intestinal disorders.

Another disability attached to such foods is that, in order to maintain the physiological needs of the body, they require to be taken in such large quantities that the carbohydrates and caloric value of the dietaries become very excessive. Thus, in the three

* Scientific Memoirs, Government of India, No. 48, p. 131.
† Ibid., No. 48, p. 54.

examples given above, the carbohydrates averaged 628·7 grammes, and the heat value 3,312 calories, which, for the average weight of the prisoners, works out at over 60 calories per kilo of body weight.

It is probable the explanation of the low percentages of nitrogen absorption shown by barley, bajra, and juar is that the proteins of these cereals do not exist in forms capable of absorption. If this explanation should turn out to be the true one, it would account for the great loss of protein in the fæces with dietaries into whose composition any of these cereals enters at all largely. Whatever the true explanation may be, these foodstuffs, so far as their protein content is concerned, exhibit a very poor degree of absorption; so much, indeed, is this the case that they are quite unsuitable to act as principals in the formation of dietaries.

The last class of food materials that it will be necessary to discuss is that derived from the Leguminosæ. The different legumens used as food include the following dals :

Arhar dal (*Cajanus indicus*).
Massur dal (*Erbum lens*).
Gram dal (*Cicer arietinum*).
Mung dal (*Phaseolus mungo*).
Mattar dal (*Pisum sativum*).
Kalai dal (*Phaseolus radiatus*).
Urid dal (*Phaseolus radiatus*).

These dals all resemble the European pea in appearance, but vary considerably in size. They are chiefly characterized by their richness in protein, being termed for this reason " the poor man's beef." The chemical composition of the different dals shows the protein content to be uniformly high, the carbohydrates well represented, and fats as a rule low in amount, although gram dal has a very high percentage of fat :

Foodstuffs.	Protein.	Carbohydrates.	Fat.
	Per Cent.	Per Cent.	Per Cent.
Mung dal	23·62	53·45	2·69
Massur dal	25·47	55·03	3·00
Gram dal	19·91	54·22	4·34
Kalai dal	22·58	58·02	1·10
Mattar dal	22·01	53·97	1·96
Arhar dal	21·70	54·06	2·50
Urid dal	22·33	55·22	1·95

As a source of nitrogen these legumens in the dietaries of the people of the East play a very important part, and take the place of animal food to a considerable extent. They are extensively used all over India and the tropics, and one member, the soy bean, has been employed for centuries by the Chinese and Japanese in the manufacture of food preparations. Taking the different countries together, they rank next to wheat and maize in importance among vegetable foods, and as a source of protein are superior to most of the cereals.

The chief protein of the pulses is legumin, which possesses the property of uniting with salts of lime, and the compound so formed is insoluble in water. Pulses should, therefore, never be cooked in hard water, unless the lime in the water has been precipitated by the addition of bicarbonate of soda. " Some of the protein of pulses exists in the form of nitrogen compounds which are not albuminoid—which are not flesh-formers, in fact— and which, for all we know, may be entirely without nutritive value. These bodies are simpler in constitution than the albuminoids, and are often of the nature of alkaloids—lupinine, a bitter basic substance from lupines is one of these ; asparagine is another. But the quantity of nitrogen existing in the pulse in the form of non-albuminoid compounds of all kinds is small, not exceeding 3 to 5 per cent. of the total albuminoids in the common kinds of ripe pulse ; in the seeds, stems, and pods of the unripe plants it is very much larger."*

Pulses are prepared in India for food in different ways ; occasionally they are ground to meal, and the meal baked with the cereal into bread of the unleavened type ; more often they are boiled in water into a form of porridge or thin gruel, and used as a sauce with the bread and vegetables. Some forms, as gram dal, are parched and eaten dry. As will be shown later, the method of cooking pulses makes a considerable difference in the absorbability of the protein element, and probably also on the carbohydrate and fat absorption. When cooked, dal, in whatever form, takes up a large quantity of water, usually about three and a half times its own weight. This increase in water means a corresponding increase in bulk, which may affect seriously the absorption of protein when the dal is given in large quantities, or when it is combined with a cereal, such as rice, that is of a bulky nature.

* Church, " Food Grains of India."

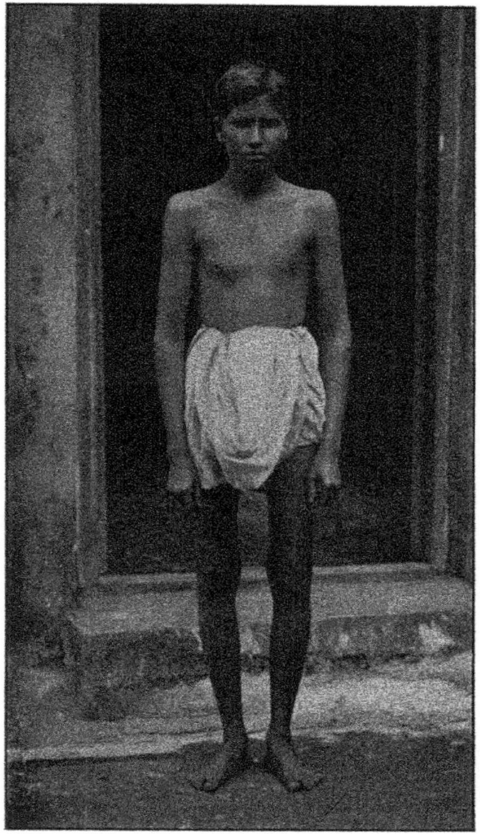

(a.) BENGALI. 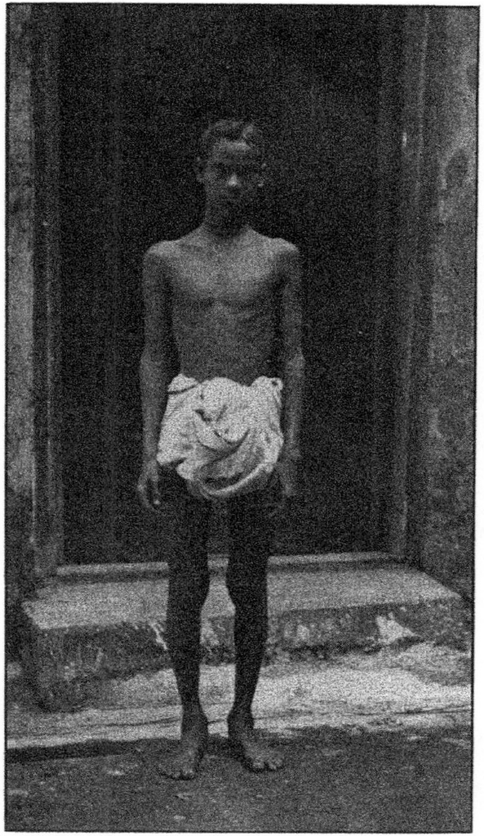   (b.) OORIYA. 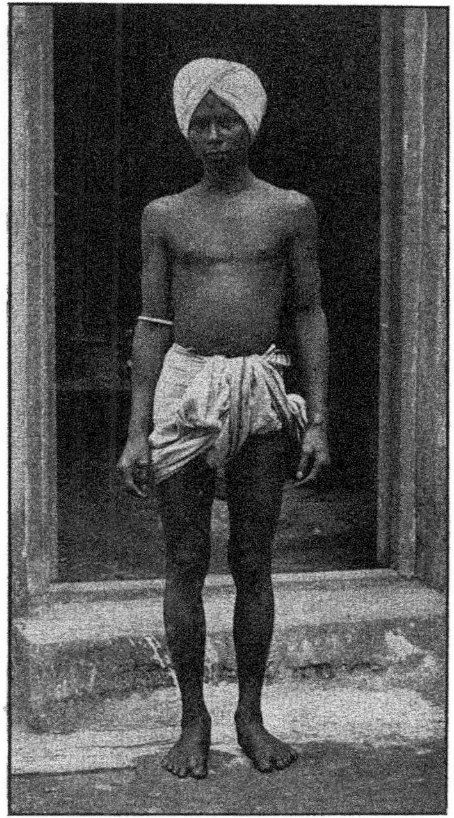   (c.) OORIYA.

Considering the importance of the pulses as food materials, up to within recent years comparatively few investigations had been made into the absorption of their several constituents. Hofman,* in 1869, reported, as the result of some experiments, that 47 per cent. of the protein of a diet of bread, lentils, and potatoes was excreted, as compared with a loss of 18 per cent. of meat protein eaten by the same person. Strumpell,* experimenting with lentils soaked in water and cooked in the usual manner, found about 40 per cent. of the protein excreted, whilst investigations into the absorption of pea and lentil flour, properly cooked, showed that under 10 per cent. of the protein is lost in the fæces. Rubner* made experiments with dried hulled peas, cooked for two or three hours, until soft, and then passed through a sieve. When large quantities were eaten he found an absorption of—

Protein	72 per cent.
Carbohydrates	93 ,,
Fat	25 ,,
Ash	64 ,,

with smaller quantities about 83 per cent. of the protein was absorbed. Malfatti,* Richter,* and Prausnitz* obtained somewhat similar results, and the important point was demonstrated that lentils are more thoroughly digested and absorbed when cooked in distilled water than when hard water is used.

Oshima,* in Japanese investigations, found the coefficient of digestibility for protein was 65 per cent., and that for carbohydrates 86 per cent. Snyder,† experimenting with legumes when eaten in combination with other foods in an ordinary mixed diet, obtained very uniform results for the different subjects under observation; the absorption of protein was found to be 80 per cent., and carbohydrates 96 per cent.

Later investigations by Wait‡ carried out on a large scale under more normal conditions—*i.e.*, the quantity of pulses not excessive, and given in an ordinary mixed diet, have extended our knowledge of the nutritive value of the pulses very considerably. The averages of the results obtained are given in the table on p. 60.

* Quoted by Wait, U.S. Department of Agriculture, Bulletin No. 187.
† Minnesota Station, Bulletin No. 92.
‡ Wait, *loc. cit.*

Character of Diet.	Digestibility of Total Diet.			Digestibility of Legumes.	
	Protein per Cent.	Fat per Cent.	Carbohydrates per Cent.	Protein per Cent.	Carbohydrates per Cent.
Basal ration	91	95	98	—	—
Basal ration and kidney beans	78	89	95	77	94
Basal ration and white beans	81	88	95	78	96
Basal ration and cow peas, whippoorwill	77	91	92	70	87
Basal ration and cow peas, clag	81	93	94	74	88
Basal ration and cow peas, lady	87	91	97	83	95

It is evident from these results that the legumes experimented with are somewhat less thoroughly digested than other common food materials, and that the addition of the legumes to the basal diet caused a lowering of the percentages of absorption.

In investigating the nutritive value of the Indian dals two factors were found to affect seriously the absorption of protein. One of these was the bulk of the basal diets, and another was the large quantities of the dals given in some of the gaol dietaries. With regard to the latter point, it has been the favourite method of raising the nitrogenous element, without increasing the carbonaceous, to give large quantities of the pulses in these vegetable dietaries which would be otherwise deficient in protein. Thus, in the gaols of the United Provinces, dal in quantities of over 8 ounces enters into the composition of some of the dietetic combinations sanctioned for prisoners. In such cases the protein absorption from the diets was found to be very poor, and the amount of nitrogen in the fæces exceedingly high.

An example* will make this clear.

Five prisoners were kept on the following diet for five days, the fæces for the period separated in the usual manner, and the nitrogen content determined:

Juar	22 ozs. presenting	7·4844 grms. of nitrogen.
Urid dal	6 ,, ,,	6·2940 ,, ,,
Arhar dal	2 ,, ,,	1·9964 ,, ,,
Vegetables	6 ,, ,,	0·5000 ,, ,,

Of a total intake of 16·2748 grammes of nitrogen, only 8·9992 grammes were absorbed, or 55·3 per cent. of the nitrogen offered in the diet. The fæces gave 7·2756 grammes of nitrogen per man daily.

* Scientific Memoirs, Government of India, No. 48, p. 43.

It will be noticed that over half of the nitrogen of this diet is derived from the pulses, which is beyond the percentage from which the maximum protein absorption will be obtained. From the coefficients of digestibility worked out for the different foodstuffs present in this diet, over 60 per cent. of its nitrogen should have been absorbed, so that the excessive quantities of pulse cause decrease in the actual and relative absorption of its protein element.

In connection with this point Church states : "The digestibility of the albuminoids in pulse as compared with that of the corresponding compounds in the cereals has usually been regarded as low. In general, they are not only digested and absorbed at a slower rate, but a larger proportion of the total amount present remains unattacked and unused in its passage through the alimentary canal. The proportion of unused to used albuminoids is proportionately highest when the pulse forms the largest part of the ration ; it is much reduced when the pulse constitutes not more than one-fourth of the daily food."* It was found in dealing with the gaol dietaries of Bengal and the United Provinces that it was useless to increase the quantity of pulse beyond an average of 5 ounces per man daily. Larger quantities than this seem to act more as an irritant than as a food, and have a decided tendency to set up diarrhœa, thus seriously deteriorating the value of the diet.

In dietaries where the pulse is improperly cooked—as, for instance, is the case in the method of parching gram dal—it is probable that a large proportion of the contained nutriment never comes into thorough contact with the digestive juices, and passes out in the fæces practically unchanged. Gram dal, on this account partly at least, showed the poorest percentage of protein absorption of all the pulses investigated. With regard to the other factor that was found to affect the protein absorption from the pulses—viz., the total bulk of the diet—experiments carried out with the voluminous rice dietaries of Bengal prisoners showed that it was futile to increase the nitrogen intake by the addition of pulse beyond a certain optimum quantity, in the hope of obtaining an augmented protein absorption.

From actual observations† it was demonstrated that, with a constant intake of nitrogen derived from rice, but with a varying

---

* Church, "Food Grains of India."
† Scientific Memoirs, Government of India, No. 37, pp. 66-71.

intake of nitrogen derived from dal, no increase in nitrogenous metabolism accompanied an augmentation of the nitrogen presented in the form of pulse. Thus—

Batches of five men under observation for five days on each separate diet :

```
Nitrogen of      ⎧ N. of arhar dal  .. 150·10 grms. showed 196·25 grms. absorbed.
rice and       + ⎪ N. of massur dal     188·40   ,,      ,,   198·60   ,,       ,,
vegetables       ⎨ N. of massur dal     171·30   ,,      ,,   198·13   ,,       ,,
constant.        ⎩ N. of mung dal  .. 160·81     ,,      ,,   193·54   ,,       ,,
```

Other results were found to corroborate the above finding. Thus—

Diets Investigated.	Grammes of Nitrogen Absorbed.	Per Cent. of Nitrogen of Diet Absorbed.
Burma rice .. 20 ozs. ⎫ + ⎧ Massur dal.. 6 ozs.	8·12	56·87
Vegetables .. 6 ,, ⎭ ⎩ ,, ,, .. 5 ,,	8·06	61·97
Country rice .. 26 ozs. ⎫ + ⎧ Mung dal .. 6 ozs.	7·49	51·34
Vegetables .. 6 ,, ⎭ ⎩ ,, ,, .. 7 ,,	7·42	47·61

A large number of feeding experiments have been made on Indian prisoners to determine the protein absorption from some of the more common pulses in use. So long as the same sample of dal was adhered to, very uniform results were obtained ; but samples of the same pulses sometimes showed considerable variations in protein content in the several gaols where investigations were carried out, so that an accompanying variation in the coefficient of protein absorption was only to be expected. As in the case of wheat, it was only with difficulty that good clean samples of the several dals could be obtained, the usual condition met with being a mixture of several varieties, and in the ordinary gaol stock other types of seeds occurred that did not belong to the lentils at all. Thus, the results[*] obtained for the absorption of protein in the different gaols were—

BENARES GAOL.

```
Protein absorption from gram dal   ..  No. 27 shows 61·8 per cent.
      ,,          ,,       ,,         ,, ,,  28  ,,   60·9    ,,
      ,,          ,,       ,,   arhar dal and ⎫ ,, 28 ,, 84·1 ,,
                                    vegetables ⎭
      ,,          ,,       ,,   arhar dal and ⎫ ,, 39 ,, 84·0 ,,
                                    vegetables ⎭
```

---

[*] Scientific Memoirs, Indian Government, No. 48. Numbers refer to the experiments.

Naini Gaol.

Protein absorption from gram dal .. No. 62a shows 65·9 per cent.
,, ,, ,, ,, ,, ,, 62b ,, 65·5 ,,
,, ,, ,, arhar dal and vegetables } ,, 55a ,, 83·8 ,,
,, ,, ,, arhar dal and vegetables } ,, 55b ,, 83·8 ,,
,, ,, ,, urid dal ,, 56 ,, 69·2 ,,

Lucknow Gaol.

Protein absorption from gram dal .. No. 69 shows 66·8 per cent.
,, ,, ,, ,, ,, ,, 70 ,, 65·7 ,,
,, ,, ,, ,, ,, ,, 71 ,, 68·2 ,,
,, ,, ,, arhar dal and vegetables { ,, 63 / ,, 64 / ,, 66 } ,, 80·6 ,,
,, ,, ,, arhar dal { ,, 63 / ,, 66 } ,, 81·2 ,,

Agra Gaol.

Protein absorption from gram dal .. { No. 77 / ,, 78 / ,, 80 / ,, 83 } shows 62·9 per cent.
,, ,, ,, arhar dal ,, 91 ,, 73·6 ,,
,, ,, ,, arhar dal and vegetables } ,, 82 ,, 73·6 ,,
,, ,, ,, arhar dal and vegetables } ,, 95 ,, 73·8 ,,
,, ,, ,, urid dal and vegetables { ,, 85 / ,, 86 / ,, 88 } ,, 54·3 ,,

The lowest figures were obtained in experiments on prisoners in Agra Gaol, not only for the protein absorption from the pulses, but also for that of the cereals. The explanation of this was the more than ordinary contamination of the foodstuffs, and also, in the case of the pulses, the very large quantities of these materials that were given in the dietaries. An examination of the experiments, Nos. 85, 86, 88, and 91, from which the absorption is very poor, shows that about 50 per cent. of the total nitrogen of the diets is derived from pulses, and there can be little doubt but that the quantity of these foodstuffs from which the best absorption is obtained has been passed. Thus—

No. 85.

Wheat	..	14 ozs.	presents	6·3504 grms. N.	A total intake of nitrogen per man daily of 17·5324 grms.
Juar	..	10 ,,	,,	3·4020 ,,	
Urid dal	..	4 ,,	,,	4·1960 ,,	
Gram dal	..	4 ,,	,,	3·0840 ,,	
Vegetables		6 ,,	,,	0·5000 ,,	

Of this only 10·2509 grammes nitrogen were absorbed, or 58·4 per cent. of the total nitrogen offered in the diet; 7·2815 grammes nitrogen were recovered from the fæces.

No. 86.

Wheat	10 ozs.	presents	4·5360 grms. N.	A total intake of nitrogen per man daily of 15·718 grms.
Juar	10 ,,	,,	3·4020 ,,	
Urid dal	4 ,,	,,	4·1960 ,,	
Gram dal	4 ,,	,,	3·0840 ,,	
Vegetables	6 ,,	,,	0·5000 ,,	

Of this only 9·106 grammes nitrogen were absorbed, or 57·9 per cent. of the total nitrogen offered in the diet; 6·612 grammes nitrogen were recovered from the fæces.

No. 88.

Wheat	10 ozs.	presents	4·5360 grms. N.	A total intake of nitrogen per man daily of 17·0788 17·0788 grms.
Juar	14 ,,	,,	4·7628 ,,	
Urid dal	4 ,,	,,	4·1960 ,,	
Gram dal	4 ,,	,,	3·0840 ,,	
Vegetables	6 ,,	,,	0·5000 ,,	

Of this only 9·8038 grammes nitrogen were absorbed, or 55·9 per cent. of the total nitrogen offered in the diet; 7·275 grammes nitrogen were recovered from the fæces.

No. 91.

Juar	22 ozs.	presents	7·4844 grms. N.	A total intake of nitrogen per man daily of 16·2748 grms.
Urid dal	6 ,,	,,	6·2940 ,,	
Arhar dal	2 ,,	,,	1·9964 ,,	
Vegetables	6 ,,	,,	0·5000 ,,	

Of this only 8·9992 grammes nitrogen were absorbed, or 55·3 per cent. of the total nitrogen offered in the diet; 7·2756 grammes nitrogen were recovered from the fæces.

These results are sufficient to show how very inferior the absorption of nitrogen is from diets of a type in which the main source of protein is the pulses—*i.e.*, diets in which the other constituents being poor in protein, an effort is made to bring the diet up to the normal protein standard by increasing the quantity of pulses to an excessive degree. The effect of large quantities of pulse is not only to cause a decrease in the percentage of protein absorption from the pulses themselves, but also to lessen the degree of protein absorption from the other constituents of the diet. In Agra Gaol the amount of pulses entering into the composition of the diets experimented with was too high, practically never less than 7 ounces, and often over 8 ounces; this would account for—partially at least—the lower coefficients of absorbability obtained for the foodstuffs investigated in that gaol. On the other hand, the wheat was of poor quality, containing a large percentage of barley and other contaminating factors, so that a high level of nitrogenous metabolism could not be expected from diets made up of poor wheat and excessive quantities of pulses.

Selecting the results obtained for the coefficients of digestibility where the foodstuffs were of fair quality and where the amount of any individual food material, such as the pulses, was not excessive, the following may be accepted as representing the average coefficients of digestibility for the Indian cereals and pulses investigated :

Food Materials.	Coefficient of Protein Absorbability.	Coefficient of Carbohydrate Absorbability.
	Per Cent.	Per Cent.
First quality of wheat	80·6	—
Ordinary wheat	70·3	96·5
Arhar dal with vegetables	82·8	92·3
Arhar dal	86·5	96·8
Mung dal	85·6	—
Gram dal	64·9	97·7
Urid dal	69·2	..
Barley	57·6	96·0
Juar	53·6	97·8
Bajra	49·4	—
Vegetables	76·3	—

In the experimental work necessary for the determination of these coefficients, the aim ever kept in view was to maintain the characteristics of a normal well-balanced diet. In no instances were large quantities of any one food material added, as seems to be the usual custom in investigations of this nature, so that the coefficient of absorbability presented above are such as would be likely to hold good for the protein and carbohydrate constituents of the foodstuffs when consumed in ordinary quantities, and not those obtained when some one food material is given out of all proportion to what would ever be the case except under artificial or experimental conditions.

It has already been pointed out that the ordinary wheat supplied to the gaols is mixed to a considerable extent with barley and other grains. This accounts for the much lower coefficient of protein absorption obtained for ordinary wheat than that shown by wheat of good quality—a difference of just over 10 per cent. The gram dal was investigated under conditions that were not conducive to a high degree of protein absorption ; it was eaten in the form of parched gram, practically not cooked at all, and retaining all its cellulose and other elements, a certain amount of moisture alone having been got rid of. Strumpell showed long since under such conditions, when pulses are not given in a state of fine division and when badly cooked, that the loss of protein may rise to 40 per cent. However, parching was the customary method of preparing gram dal for consumption, and it was therefore desirable to detérmine the protein and carbohydrate absorption under local conditions. Over a large number of observations the protein absorption was never found to fall below 61 per cent., the average working out at 65 per cent.

Of all the varieties of dal experimented with, arhar dal was found to give the highest coefficient of protein absorption. Under favourable conditions, when combined with first quality of wheat, over 86 per cent. of its protein is taken up by the intestinal tract. This variety is the favourite form of dal with the wheat-eating population of India, and it is quite probable, in the light of Pawlow's investigations, that the desire for this food material is a factor that must be taken into consideration in any explanation of the high degree of protein absorption shown by arhar dal. Although it was impossible to obtain uniform results for the absorption of the protein of the foodstuffs in the bulky dietaries of Bengal gaols, when the volume of these diets was decreased to rational proportions, the coefficient of protein digestibility of arhar dal worked out to be practically identical with that given in the above table.* Under similar conditions of decreased bulk the absorption of the protein of mung dal—the favourite form with the rice-eating Bengali— was found to be on the average about 85 per cent.†

With regard to the other varieties of the pulses, massur, kalai, and mattar dals, no exact figures representing the percentages of protein absorption could be determined, as these varieties were only used in the bulky rice dietaries of the Bengal gaols. None of them appeared to give as good results as arhar and mung dals, but without experiments under conditions where the volume of the dietaries is such as the stomach can successfully cope with, it is not possible to determine accurately the degree of protein absorption. These dals are not made use of in the less bulky wheat diets of the United Provinces.

* Scientific Memoirs, Government of India, No. 37, p. 147.   † *Ibid.*, p. 149.

CHAPTER IV

THE PROTEIN METABOLISM OF MANKIND

HAVING surveyed in general terms some of the food materials extensively used in different countries, and having examined their gross chemical composition and the averages of the percentage absorption of their proximate principles, we shall now take into consideration the dietaries of mankind in general, and discuss the nutritive requirements and the extent of nitrogenous interchange attained by the various peoples concerning whom information is available.

In his introductory remarks on the general principles of dietetics Sir Lauder Brunton states: "The subject of food is one upon which countless experiments have been made by myriads of men during thousands and perhaps millions of years. In all parts of the world, from prehistoric times until now, men have been constantly engaged in finding out what things were good to eat and what things they had better avoid." It is only, however, within comparatively recent times that the study of dietetics has been accurately pursued and placed on a scientific footing. Students of nutrition from different parts of the world have laid their contributions at the feet of Knowledge, and Wisdom and Understanding are gradually emerging from darkness into light.

Japan, Russia, and the different European countries, have all made valuable additions in the advances recorded, but, at the present time, to none do we owe the same debt as to America for the stimulating influence of her many workers in this field, and for the exceedingly valuable contributions they have made to the scientific pursuit of the principles of proper feeding.

In the following pages it will be found necessary to make reference to many of those engaged in this line of research, as, for instance, Atwater, Langworthy, Benedict, Folin, etc., in America; Zuntz, Ranke, Pflüger, v. Noorden, and others, in Germany; but it is only meet that special mention should be made of Chittenden, who, in first stirring the nutritional pool by the publication of his two well-known volumes, has done more to awaken interest, stimulate research, and lift the subject of dietetics from the playground of quacks and charlatans, than perhaps any of his predecessors. That good will eventually accrue from the extensive investigations that have followed on the publication of Chittenden's studies cannot be doubted, and it may be hoped that before long the whole subject of dietetics and food requirements may be lifted out of the vale of empiricism, in which it has hitherto lain, and raised to one of those pinnacles of fame reserved for the exact sciences.

Dietary Standards.

Many different methods have been employed in the determination of the gross amount of food consumed *per capita* of the people of different countries. A rough average may be obtained from a statistical survey of the amount of food materials available—certain factors for waste being taken into consideration—this amount divided by the total population will give a figure which represents a general average, but which is of little use where anything approaching accuracy is demanded. Russell[*] has collected a great mass of information on the foodstuffs, diets, and physical characteristics of different races and nations which, although of great interest from many standpoints, is not sufficiently detailed to be of any great service in arriving at the quantities of the proximate principles present in the different dietaries.

A more accurate method of obtaining the desired information is by means of what has been termed dietary studies; in these individuals, or groups of individuals, are kept under observation, the total food consumed is carefully recorded, samples analyzed, and the value of the dietaries in protein, carbohydrates, and fat computed. This method may be undertaken when there is free selection of food, or, as in public institutions, where the choice of food is limited.

More accurate methods are those where the subjects under observation are placed under suitable conditions for the analyses of the food and excreta over a stated period; again, there may be free choice of food, or, if the intention is to study the effects of different food materials, the choice may be limited. The most laborious, but at the same time the most accurate, method

[*] Russell, "Strength and Diet," London, 1905.

is that of the respiration calorimeter, in which the total heat generated in the body under different conditions, the waste products, work done, etc., are measured and expressed in terms of heat. The amount of potential energy to be supplied in the form of food in order to maintain body equilibrium can be computed from the heat given off from the body under the different experimental conditions. By means of certain known factors this required energy can be expressed as so much protein, carbohydrates, and fat.

By means of these and other methods of statistical and experimental study a fairly accurate knowledge has been obtained of the amounts of protein, carbohydrates, fat, and energy ordinarily consumed by people of different classes and in different countries. The knowledge thus derived has led to the general acceptance of certain standards for the average food consumption of different classes, and has brought out this fact: " That all over the world people who can obtain such food as they desire use liberal rather than small quantities; and that the more active or severe the work done, the larger the quantity of food eaten."[*]

The standards that have been most widely accepted, such as those of Voit, Atwater, Rubner, and others, all agree pretty closely in the quantities of their constituents with the average dietaries to which custom and instinct have guided mankind in the formation of his dietetic habits. These standards have been generally regarded as representing the minimum amount necessary for the maintenance of the average man, under average conditions, doing a moderate amount of work, in health and strength. Some of these standards are—

	Protein.	Carbohydrate.	Fat.	Heat Value.
	Grammes.	Grammes.	Grammes.	Calories.
Ranke	100	240	100	2,324
Munk	105	500	56	3,022
Voit	118	500	56	3,055
Rubner	127	509	52	3,092
Moleschott	130	550	40	3,160
Atwater	125	400	125	3,315

It will be observed that there is a general consensus of opinion that the protein element should amount to over 100 grammes a day, and that the energy value should be over 3,000 calories.

[*] Benedict, "The Nutritive Requirements of the Body," *American Journal of Physiology*, 1906, xvi.

Benedict,* by taking into account the large amount of data available as a result of dietary studies in different countries, gives the following estimates of the average food consumption of people under certain circumstances:

Subjects.	Protein. Total.	Protein. Digestible.	Fuel Value.
	Grammes.	Grammes.	Calories.
People with active muscular work, such as lumbermen, athletes, etc.	175	160	5,500
People with ordinary muscular work, such as carpenters, farmers, labourers, etc.	115	105	3,300
People with light muscular work, such as professional and business men, clerks, etc.	100	92	2,700

A selection of some of the available data is here presented. A large number of results obtained from dietary studies have been collected, but it would not serve any useful purpose to go into a mass of details. Taking the results as a whole, they conform very closely to the standard dietaries already shown:

Subjects.	Protein.	Heat Value.
	Grammes.	Calories.
Teamsters, marble-workers, etc., with hard labour, Boston, U.S.	254	7,804
Brewery labourers, Munich, very severe work	223	5,692
Brickmakers, U.S.	222	6,464
Swedish workmen	189	4,726
Lumbermen, U.S.	185	6,400
Weavers, England	151	3,475
Average dietary of five halls of residence for students in Edinburgh	143	3,979
Dietary of a students' club in Finland	157	3,984
Medical students, Sweden	127	2,723
Chinese laundrymen, U.S.	135	3,480
Professor, Japan	123	2,343
Average of twenty-one dietary studies amongst the labouring classes in Dublin	98·5	3,117
Chinese dentist's family	115	2,705
Russian workmen	132	3,675
Average diet of a labourer's family in Edinburgh	107·7	3,228
Poor families in New York	75	2,087
Students, Japan	97	2,343

* Benedict, *loc. cit.*

It would therefore appear that in the different countries where dietary studies have been carried out, those who have a free choice of food arrange to eat such quantities as shall permit of at least 100 grammes of protein intake daily. It is uncommon to find much below this figure except in conditions of poverty; thus factory girls in Leipsic and sewing girls in London earning poor wages have been shown to live on diets yielding little over 50 grammes of protein and less than 2,000 calories of total energy. When muscular work is excessive or fatiguing, there is a great demand for a high caloric and protein value of the diet. This is recognized in the framing of the army rations of the different nations in peace and war:

CALORIC VALUE OF RATIONS.*

Army Rations.	Peace.	War.
Great Britain: Regulation diet	2,946	3,987
Actual diet obtained	3,319	
Germany	2,592	small, 3,613 / large, 4,213
France	2,310	small, 3,079 / large, 3,413

The requirements of the body for increased protein and energy during severe muscular exertion is well exemplified in Atwater's standards, which embody the results of modern investigations into the diet of adults under different conditions:

Subjects.	Protein.	Calories.
Women with light muscular exercise	90	2,400
Women with moderate muscular work	100	2,700
Man without muscular work	100	2,700
Man with light muscular work	112	3,000
Man with moderate muscular work	125	3,500
Man with hard muscular work	150	4,500

Taking the average weight of Europeans and Americans at 68 to 70 kilos, or about 11 stone, the standard dietary for a man doing a moderate amount of work should offer 1·4 to 1·7 grammes of protein and 40 calories per kilo of body weight.

Turning now from dietaries of the European and American type, on which an immense amount of work has been done, let

* Spriggs, "Sutherland's System of Diet and Dietetics." London, 1908.

us examine the results that have been obtained with dietaries peculiar to Japan, India, and the tropics.

Oshima,* in his digest of Japanese investigation on the nutrition of man, gives the results of a large number of dietary studies. Although these do not deal with the poorer classes or rural population to any great extent, he has succeeded in collecting a valuable amount of information on the foodstuffs and dietaries of the Japanese. He shows that soldiers and sailors, and those in comfortable circumstances in other classes, including professional and business men and students, are in general well nourished. The amounts of protein and energy in the diet of these classes compare well with those in the diet of people under similar circumstances in Europe and America, especially when allowance is made for the smaller average weight of the Japanese.

The dietary studies with the poorer classes, including employees, prisoners, military colonists, and investigations on purely vegetarian diets, show that the amount of protein is about 60 grammes per man daily and the energy about 2,500 calories. The average body weight of the Japanese is computed to be about 54 kilos; this would mean a metabolism of 1·111 grammes protein or 0·177 grammes of nitrogen per kilo of body weight, as contrasted with 0·224 to 0·27 grammes nitrogen per kilo of body weight in Europeans and Americans.

The amount of animal food in the Japanese dietaries is much less than in the average American dietary. A comparison is given of the total protein derived from an animal and other sources in 25 Japanese and 185 American studies:

Dietary Studies.	Total Animal Protein per Cent.	Cereals per Cent.	Legumes per Cent.	Vegetables per Cent.
25 Japanese studies	38·0	47·5	8·2	6·3
185 American ,,	61·2	30·5	2·0	6·3

A special characteristic of the Japanese diet, and also, to some extent, of Indian dietaries, is that the amount of fat is very low; in Japan, also, dairy products are practically unknown. In connection with the commonly accepted idea that the Japanese are vegetarians, it is interesting to note that Oshima comes to much the same conclusion as that arrived at in discussing the

* Oshima, U.S. Department of Agriculture, Bulletin No. 159.

food habits of the people of India—viz., that they are vegetarians from force of adverse financial circumstances rather than from principle, and, except in the case of a relatively small number of strict adherents to Buddhism, they eat animal food whenever it can be afforded.

Another misconception that Oshima refers to is the popular belief that rice is the principal, if not practically the only, food of the large majority of the Japanese and other Oriental people. As has already been pointed out in connection with Indian foodstuffs, rice is only cheap in those parts of the East where the conditions necessary for its cultivation are favourable, particularly where the rainfall is abundant. In Japan, as in India, though rice is a very important article of diet, and is eaten in relatively large quantities where it can be afforded, it is by no means the only food material, nor is it in all cases the principal cereal. In large tracts of India, away from the coast-line, rice hardly enters into the dietaries of the people, being too expensive for regular consumption, and is only used on special occasions as a luxury. The proportion of total nutrients of the Japanese diets supplied by rice Oshima gives as follows :

Dietary Studies.	Proportion of Total Nutrients supplied by Rice.		
	Protein.	Fat.	Carbohydrates.
Average 24 studies	Per Cent. 53·2	Per Cent. 23·0	Per Cent. 89·5
,, 9 ,, (Navy)	21·5	10·4	52·1

From statistics collated by the Department of Agriculture and Commerce, Tokyo, showing the proportions of the different vegetable foods consumed by the Japanese in 1880, the following averages were derived as applicable to the country as a whole :

Rice	.. 53·00	per cent.
Barley and wheat	.. 27·00	,,
Millets, buckwheat, legumes, etc.	.. 13·90	,,
Tubers and other vegetables ..	.. 6·00	,,
Fruits	.. 0·05	,,
Sea algæ	.. 0·05	,,

So that cereals other than rice form by no means an unimportant part of the whole dietary.

It will now be of interest to give summaries of the dietaries investigated in Japan, and contrast them with results of dietary studies under the same conditions as nearly as possible in America:

Dietary Studies.	Protein.	Fuel Value.
	Grammes.	Calories.
Professional and business men:		
Average of 13 studies	87	2,190
Professional men in United States:		
Average of 14 studies	104	3,220
Medical students (Japanese):		
Average of 8 studies	98	2,800
Military cadets (Japanese):		
Average of 11 studies	113	3,185
College clubs in United States:		
Average of 15 studies	107	3,580
Hard labour:		
Rice-cleaner (Japan)	110·5	4,107
Jinricksha man (Japan)	158	5,050
Coal-miner (Japan)	145	2,660
Football team (United States)	226	6,590
Japanese Army:		
Average of 261 studies	124	3,360
Japanese Navy:		
Revised (1900) allowance, peace	151	3,250
American Navy	145	4,280

With regard to the army ration, when the weight of the soldiers, which is undoubtedly less than that of European troops, is taken into account, it will be seen to compare very favourably with the protein content and energy value of the dietaries of the British Army. Thus—

Army Rations.	Protein.	Fuel Value.
	Grammes.	Calories.
Average food supplied gratis to four British regiments	133	3,369
British soldiers in detention, without hard labour	127	3,272
British Army minimum war ration (South Africa)	138	3,903
Russian Army war ration (Manchuria)	187	4,891
Japanese Army war ration (Manchuria)	158	4,343

It is evident from these figures, supplied by the Committee on the Physiological Effects of Food, Training, and Clothing on the Soldier, that in proportion to their respective body weights the Japanese were more abundantly fed than the Russian soldier in Manchuria or the British in South Africa.

We may now refer in detail to the dietary study Oshima records with a jinricksha man, as its counterpart will be found when we come to examine the dietary of the dandy carriers of Darjeeling. This man was thirty-three years old, and weighed 62·4 kilos. His work was very laborious, and consisted in drawing his ricksha with one man in it anything from fifteen to thirty miles daily. The ricksha men often run long distances with heavy passengers ; a not uncommon run is from Tokyo to Nikko, a distance of sixty-eight miles, which they will cover in fifteen hours.

This is an example of those classes who are held up by vegetarians as demonstrating the wonderful results that can be obtained by a simple vegetable diet, as the usual impression conveyed is that these feats of strength and endurance have been performed on a few handfuls of boiled rice.

The diet of this man supplied 158 grammes of protein and a fuel value of 5,050 calories, and was both abundant and varied. It is particularly worthy of note that 41·1 per cent. of the total protein in the diet was derived from an animal source. Contrary to the popular belief, these jinricksha men spend a comparatively large part of their income on animal food. Tiegel states that they eat large quantities of rice during their working periods, but during the periods of rest they consume large amounts of fish, eggs, beef, and pork. He states that there has been a considerable degree of misrepresentation with regard to the amount of protein in the diet of these people.

The class in India corresponding to the jinricksha man of Japan was found to live on a protein intake of 175 grammes, of which well over 60 per cent. is derived from an animal source— in fact, these men eat from 20 to 30 ounces of beef or mutton daily.

A comparison of the conditions met with in this Japanese jinricksha man with those found for men engaged in similar work round Darjeeling is of interest.

The Japanese metabolized 0·35 gramme nitrogen, and expended almost 81 calories per kilo of body weight. He absorbed 137·1 of the 157·6 grammes of protein offered in his diet.

It was computed that the Indian *dandy walla*—average body weight 60 kilos—metabolized 0·35 grammes nitrogen (probably too low an estimate),* and expended about 100 calories per kilo of body weight, the fuel value of his diet working out at over 6,000 calories.

* Scientific Memoirs, Government of India, No. 37, p. 216.

Reference may here be made to the very satisfactory results that followed on an increase in the supply of protein in the Japanese Navy dietary in 1884. The principal changes were the substitution of bread for a large part of the rice and a large increase in the amount of protein of animal origin.

The following statistics show the improvement in health that followed on the change of diet:

1878-1883, of 29,321 marines, 9,316, or 32·5 per cent., had beri-beri.
1884,⎫
1885,⎪
1886,⎬ of 48,275   ,,   ⎧718,⎫
1887-1889,⎭   ⎨ 41, ⎬ or 1·6 per cent., had beri-beri.
                    ⎪ 3, ⎪
                    ⎩ 3, ⎭

The proportion of other diseases was also very materially decreased. It is not to be wondered at, in the light of these results, that the problems of nutrition attracted great attention in the Navy.

INVESTIGATIONS IN INDIA.

We may now take into consideration such information as is available regarding the dietaries of the inhabitants of tropical countries, and the level of nitrogenous metabolism attained.

Study 1.—The first study* carried out was on students and servants of the Medical College, Calcutta. The aim of the investigations was to obtain some idea of the average quantities of the more important constituents present in the urine of the natives of Calcutta with whom there was free choice of food.

The only point at present necessary to consider is the elimination of nitrogen shown by these observations. Over two hundred analyses were made, and on an average the amount of nitrogen excreted in the urine was just under 6 grammes per man daily. In these observations the subjects of the inquiry had a perfectly free choice of food, and their several conditions in life corresponded in every way to that of the great majority of the population of the rice-eating inhabitants of India. The excretion of 6 grammes of nitrogen in the urine would correspond to the metabolism of 35·5 grammes of protein daily, which, even after making allowance for the elimination of metabolized nitrogen in all other secretions and excretions, would mean a very low level of nitrogenous metabolism. Accepting an average of 75 per cent. for the absorption of the protein of these dietaries, even under the most favourable circumstances, the average rice-

* Scientific Memoirs, Government of India, No. 34, p. 4.

eating Bengali does not obtain more than 55 grammes of protein in his daily food. The nitrogenous metabolism per kilo of body weight of the students and servants examined works out at 0·116 gramme; the average weight of the Bengali, based on about 30,000 weighments, being 50 to 50½ kilos.

It may be pointed out that, so far as information is available, the rice-eating Bengali lives on a poorer protein supply than any of the other races on whom investigations have been carried out. Oshima's observations on the poorer classes in Japan show that the protein metabolism they attain is higher than in the case of the Bengali. In connection with this it is worthy of note that, although the Japanese are considerably smaller in stature than the average Bengali, the average weight of the Japanese is 54 to 56 kilos, whilst that of the Bengali is only about 50 kilos.

The poorer classes in Japan metabolize 0·177 gramme of nitrogen, whilst the average Bengali shows under 0·12 gramme of nitrogen undergoing metabolism per kilo of body weight. If the relative extent of surface of the two types be taken into account, the conditions will be found to be still more favourable to the Japanese than would appear from the above comparison.

To obtain anything approaching this low level of protein exchange within the body, it is necessary to have recourse to the feeding experiments carried out by Chittenden; so that the Bengali exemplifies on a large scale the experimental conditions Chittenden had to manufacture. From the results of his investigations Chittenden states that the metabolism of 0·12 gramme of nitrogen per kilo of body weight per man daily is quite sufficient to satisfy all the demands of the body for protein.

This is a subject that will require careful consideration later in this volume; at present it is only necessary to point out that, as the Bengali practically conforms to the standard laid down by Chittenden, he should therefore exhibit those "many suggestions of improvement in bodily health, of greater efficiency in working power, and of greater freedom from disease, in a system of dietetics which aims to meet the physiological needs of the body without undue waste of energy and unnecessary drain upon the functions of digestion, absorption, excretion, and metabolism in general; a system which recognizes that the smooth running of man's bodily machinery calls for the exercise of reason and intelligence, and is not to be entrusted solely to the dictates of blind instinct or to the leadings of a capricious appetite."* None of these desirable results from the effects of a low protein dietary are to be discovered in the Bengali, and this holds, despite the fact that excessive nitrogenous interchange has in all probability never been a feature of the metabolism of the rice-eating people of Bengal.

Study 2.—A dietary study was carried out, the subjects being two medical assistants in the Physiological Department of the Medical College, Calcutta, in which a careful record was kept of the total nitrogenous intake and output. These men had a free choice of food, and the dietaries were mixed in type, although the amount of animal food was small.

The results obtained were †—

Average Nitrogen Intake.	Body Weight.	Nitrogen Output.	Nitrogen Balance.	Nitrogen per Kilo of Body Weight.
8·63 grms.	61·6 kilos	8·43 grms.	0·20 grm.	0·112 grm.
10·56 ,,	50·5 ,,	10·43 ,,	0·13 ,,	0·169 ,,

These dietaries offered 53·9 and 65·9 grammes of protein respectively in the daily food, which was as nearly as possible the ordinary amount consumed by these men from day to day. The subjects of the investigation were well educated, and were in fair circumstances, so that they were not severely handicapped by financial conditions in their choice of food. The quantity of protein available in their dietaries is very little higher than that calculated for the students and servants of the college.

Study 3.—The following different scales of dietary‡ are those ordinarily in use amongst the different classes in Bengal, according to their financial and social status :

DIET I.—CULTIVATORS.

Average Diet.	Approximate Value : Proximate Principle.	Calories.
Rice .. .. .. 20 ozs. Dal .. .. .. 1 oz. Vegetables .. .. 4 ozs. Fish .. .. .. 1 oz. Oil .. .. .. 1 ,,	Protein .. .. 52 grms. Carbohydrates .. 475 ,, Fat .. .. 25 ,,	2,390

* Chittenden, " The Nutrition of Man," p. 228.
† Scientific Memoirs, Government of India, No. 34, p. 36.
‡ Collected by Assistant-Surgeon Lal Mohan Ghosal, Physiological Department, Calcutta. " Food and Drugs." 1910.

Diet II.—Middle Classes (not above Indigence).

Average Diet.	Approximate Value: Proximate Principle.	Calories.
Rice .. .. .. 16 ozs. Dal .. .. .. 1 oz. Vegetables .. .. 4 ozs. Fish .. .. .. 1 oz. Milk .. .. .. 4 ozs. Oil .. .. .. 1 oz.	Protein .. .. 50 grms. Carbohydrates .. 400 ,, Fat .. .. .. 50 ,,	2,310

Diet III.—Middle Classes (above Indigence).

Average Diet.	Approximate Value: Proximate Principle.	Calories.
Rice .. .. .. 6 ozs. Wheat flour .. 6 ,, Dal .. .. .. 1 oz. Vegetables .. .. 4 ozs. Fish .. .. .. 2 ,, Milk .. .. .. 8 ,, Butter .. .. 1 oz. Oil .. .. .. 1 ,, Meat and eggs are also added.	Protein .. .. 70 grms. Carbohydrates .. 300 ,, Fat .. .. .. 90 ,, Protein varies with the quantity of animal material consumed	2,350

Diet IV.—Well-to-do People.

Average Diet.	Approximate Value: Proximate Principle.	Calories.
Rice .. .. .. 4 ozs. Wheat flour .. 6 ,, Dal .. .. .. ½ oz. Vegetables .. .. 4 ozs. Fish .. .. .. 4 ,, Milk .. .. .. 16 ,, Butter .. .. 4 ,, Oil .. .. .. 1 oz. Meat and eggs are eaten, also sweets freely	Protein, 85 to 100 grms., depending on the amount of meat and eggs Carbohydrates, 300 to 400 grms., depending on the amount of sweets Fat .. .. 150 grms.	2·950 to 3·450

The diet varies considerably according to the choice of food, but it may be taken as very liberal in all its elements.

DIET V.—STUDENTS LIVING IN PRIVATELY MANAGED MESS-HOUSES.

Average Diet.	Approximate Value: Proximate Principles.	Calories.
Rice .. 12 ozs. Dal .. 1 oz. Vegetables .. 4 ozs. Fish .. 2 ,, Milk .. 4 ,, Butter .. 2 ,, Oil .. 2 ,, Meat and eggs are also added, but not to a great extent	Protein .. .. 55 grms. Carbohydrates .. 325 ,, Fat .. .. 90 ,,	2,400

DIET VI.—STUDENTS IN GOVERNMENT HOSTELS.

Average Diet.	Approximate Value: Proximate Principles.	Calories.
Rice .. 16 ozs. Dal .. 2 ,, Vegetables .. 4 ,, Fish .. 1 oz. Butter .. 1 ,, Oil .. 1 ,, Meat twice a week	Protein .. .. 67 grms. Carbohydrates .. 550 ,, Fat .. .. 60 ,,	3,150

As would be expected, the protein and fat constituents of these dietaries are lowest in the cases of the poorest classes, and highest in the case of well-to-do people; while the opposite is the case in the carbohydrate element. It will be noticed that fish and milk enter into the composition of all the dietaries; even the poorest cultivator is usually able to obtain a small amount of milk daily. Fish the Bengali is particularly fond of, and, owing to the large number of rivers, tanks, pools, and nullahs, a large supply of fish is always available at a moderate price, or for the catching.

Taken in conjunction with the results obtained from the observations made on students, servants, and medical assistants, the above dietaries may be accepted as representing faithfully the average food consumption of the people of Bengal according to their particular circumstances. These dietaries have been given in full detail for two reasons: first, to show that wherever possible the Bengali prefers a mixed type of dietary to a purely vegetable kind, and that milk and fish may be taken as common articles of food even amongst the poorer classes.

The second and more important reason is to clear up a misconception into which Chittenden appears to have fallen with regard to the dietary of the mass of the people of Bengal. In his very interesting and instructive paper on the merits of a low protein dietary, read before the Therapeutic Section at the last meeting of the British Medical Association, Chittenden,* whilst admitting the poor physique of the Bengali, his lack of good health, want of vigour, and poor capacity for manual labour, and low resistance to disease and infection, attributes these characteristics not to his poor supply of protein, but to the character of the food.

In proof of this he quotes extracts from the memoirs dealing with the work done on the metabolism of the Bengali and on the gaol dietaries of Bengal. In the greater part of these extracts it was the gaol dietaries that were being criticized and not the dietary of the people in general.

The full gaol diet for Bengali prisoners is—

$$\left.\begin{array}{ll} \text{Rice} & 26 \text{ ozs.} \\ \text{Dal} & 6 \text{ ,,} \\ \text{Vegetables} & 6 \text{ ,,} \end{array}\right\} = \left\{\begin{array}{ll} \text{Protein} & 93 \text{ grms.} \\ \text{Carbohydrates } 693 \text{ ,,} \\ \text{Fat} & 30 \text{ ,,} \end{array}\right\} = 3{,}500 \text{ calories,}$$

of which only about 50 to 55 per cent. of the protein is absorbed. It is with regard to the ill-balanced proportions of this type of diet that the following criticism applies : " Simply as a means of providing fuel for the system there is a very heavy wastage, while the constant fermentation and putrefaction made possible by the copious nitrogenous residue in the alimentary canal must form a source of chronic irritation to the mucous membrane of the bowel, predisposing to intestinal catarrh, diarrhœa, etc. At the same time, the products of the putrefactive micro-organisms on absorption lower the general vitality, causing anæmia, toxæmia, and many other symptoms of ill-health." Chittenden justly asks what bearing have these results on the merits of a proper low protein intake where the diet is well balanced, and shows a reasonable degree of digestibility and availability ?

The answer is simple enough. Accepting Chittenden's criterion —the loss of nitrogen in the fæces—of an ill-balanced, non-physiological dietary, the facts obtained from a study of the people of Bengal do not support his explanation of the poor physique of the rice-eating Bengali. Thus the results obtained

* Chittenden, *British Medical Journal*, September 23, 1911, p. 661.

simply represents the average amount of the nitrogen of the urine, and that no allowance has been made for the nitrogen which has undergone metabolism, but leaves the body in other ways than in the urine, or that has been retained owing to an increase of body weight. The figures given in columns 4 and 5 are, therefore, probably too low.

By making use of the coefficients of protein absorption given these can be corrected. Taking the average for the six subjects, the figures given by Chittenden and the corrected figures would read:

Average of Figures.	Intake of Nitrogen.	Intake of Protein.	Nitrogen Metabolized.	Protein Metabolized.	Utilization of Nitrogen.
	Grms.	Grms.	Grms.	Grms.	Per Cent.
As given	12·02	75·12	9·16	57·25	88·66
Corrected	12·02	75·12	10·66	66·62	88·66

There was, therefore, on the average 1·5 grammes of nitrogen, or 9·37 grammes of protein—the difference between Chittenden's and the corrected figures—daily for each subject metabolized, and either retained within the body—the subjects all show a gain in weight—or eliminated in some other way than in the urine; probably it disappeared to some extent in both these ways.

The important point, however, from our present standpoint is the average amount of the fæcal nitrogen shown by these six subjects during the period of observation. Accepting the corrected figures as properly interpreting Chittenden's meaning, the average amount of nitrogen lost in the fæces works out to be 1·36 grammes per man daily. The importance of this lies in the fact that Chittenden attributes the poor physique of the Bengali to his "unbalanced, unphysiological ration," the criterion of which would appear to be that 1·5 grammes of its contained nitrogen passes through the intestinal tract unabsorbed; whereas the well-balanced, physiological dietary of Chittenden's six subjects, during the use of which most satisfactory results were obtained, allows 1·36 grammes of its nitrogen to pass out of the body unchanged. That a difference of 0·14 grammes of nitrogen in the daily fæces could have such far-reaching consequences is scarcely credible, or that it can constitute the difference between a well-balanced, satisfactory diet and an ill-balanced, inferior diet is absurd. In this connection we may refer to the results given by Chittenden for the excretion of nitrogen in the fæces, and the absorption of protein in the experiments on his second group of subjects—soldiers of the Hospital Corps.* The figures show that many of the individuals excreted up to 2 grammes of nitrogen per day in the fæces, and absorbed less than 75 per cent. of the total protein offered. Yet, according to Chittenden, this was a well-balanced diet. Indeed, it was on the results obtained from this and similar experiments that he has based his well-known views on economy in nutrition.

It is evident, therefore, that so far as the actual amount of nitrogenous waste is concerned, the dietary of the people of Bengal compares very favourably with that made use of by Chittenden in his prolonged experiments, and that an ill-balanced character of the Bengali ration will not explain his poor physical attainments and other characteristics of malnutrition.

Study 4.—Three diets may be included in this study : one for Bengalis in a residential Government college, and two for Anglo-Indian and Eurasian students in Government colleges. As there will be occasion to deal with the effects of these dietaries in another connection, it will be sufficient at present to record their values :

DIET I.—BENGALI STUDENTS (RESIDENTIAL COLLEGE).

Protein .. .. 67·11 grms.
Carbohydrates .. 548·73 ,,   Heat value .. 3,190 calories.
Fat .. .. .. 71·55 ,,

Of the protein element, about 13 per cent. was derived from an animal source.

DIET II.—ANGLO-INDIAN AND EURASIAN STUDENTS (RESIDENTIAL COLLEGE).

Protein .. .. 87·56 grms.
Carbohydrates .. 376·53 ,,   Heat value .. 2,415 calories.
Fat .. .. .. 54·75 ,,

Of the protein element about 55 per cent., or 48·2 grammes, was derived from an animal source.

DIET III.—ANGLO-INDIAN AND EURASIAN STUDENTS (RESIDENTIAL COLLEGE).

Protein .. .. 94·97 grms.
Carbohydrates .. 467·00 ,,   Heat value .. 2,830 calories.
Fat .. .. .. 56·20 ,,

Of the protein element about 42 per cent., or 40 grammes, was derived from an animal source.

* Chittenden, " Physiological Economy in Nutrition."

Study 5.—Dietaries of the hill-tribes of Bengal.

Very accurate information was collected on the quantity and classes of food materials consumed by these hill-men under natural conditions. The investigations carried out and the effects noted will necessitate detailed consideration in connection with the relationship of food to physical development; at present we may simply record the dietaries.

DIET I.—TIBETAN BHUTIAS, BHOTAN BHUTIAS (DANDY CARRIERS, RICKSHA MEN, AND COOLIES WHO PERFORM THE HARDEST WORK).

Protein, 175 to 200 grms. Heat value, 6,300 to 6,500 calories.

Of the protein element well over 60 per cent. is derived from an animal source. It is not uncommon to find these men eating as much as 2 pounds of meat daily. They are well paid and live generously. Physically they are splendid specimens of well-developed muscular manhood. As already mentioned, they correspond to the ricksha men of Japan, and, like them, they exhibit a great weakness for a liberal supply of food, and particularly for animal protein.

DIET II.—TIBETAN LAMAS (PRIESTS AND THOSE WHO HAVE NOT SUCH HARD WORK AS THE DANDY CARRIERS).

Protein, 160 to 180 grms. Heat value, 4,000 to 4,250 calories.

DIET III.—GENERAL DIET OF THE MORE POORLY-FED CLASSES WHO EARN LOWER WAGES.

Protein, 150 to 160 grms. Heat value, 3,250 to 3,500 calories.

DIET IV.—DIET OF SIKHIM BHUTIAS (HARD-WORKING CLASSES).

Protein, 130 to 140 grms. Heat value, 3,200 to 3,300 calories.

DIET V.—DIET OF LEPCHAS (POORER CLASSES OF SIKHIM BHUTIAS).

Protein, 112 to 125 grms. Heat value, 3,500 to 3,800 calories.

In all these dietaries a large part of the protein comes from beef or mutton, up to 70 per cent., except in Diet V., the poorer classes of Lepchas not being able to afford more than $\frac{1}{2}$ pound of meat daily, which provides about 50 per cent. of the total protein of their dietary. Rice also enters more largely into the diet of the Lepchas.

DIET VI.—DIET OF THE NEPALESE CHUTTRIES.

Protein, 120 to 130 grms., of which less than 40 per cent. is derived from an animal source.

PLATE

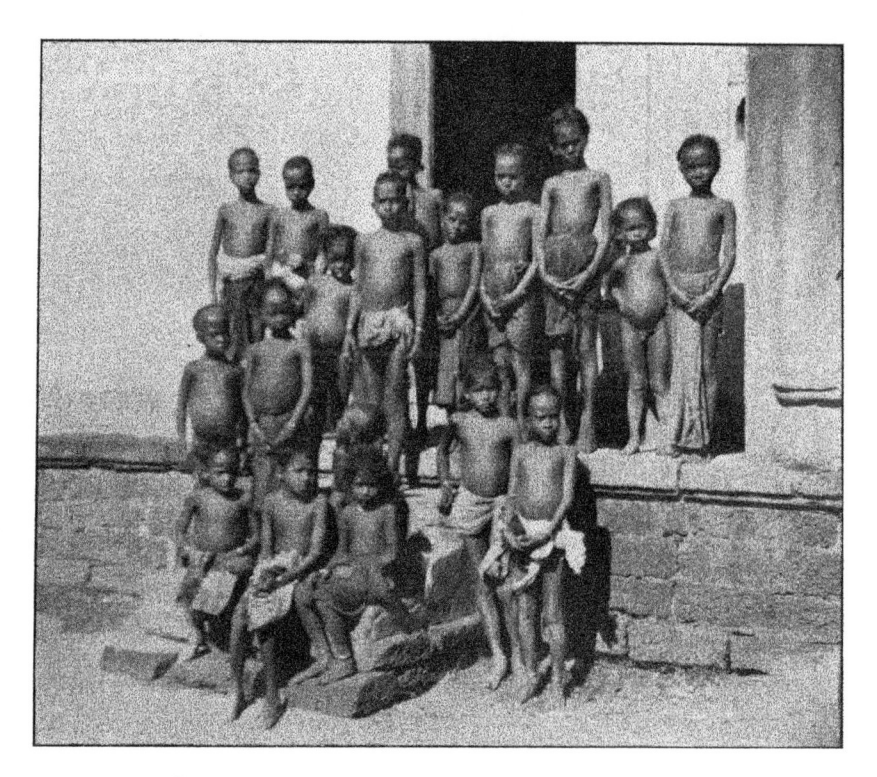

(*a.*) A GROUP OF RICE-EATING OORIYA CHILDREN.

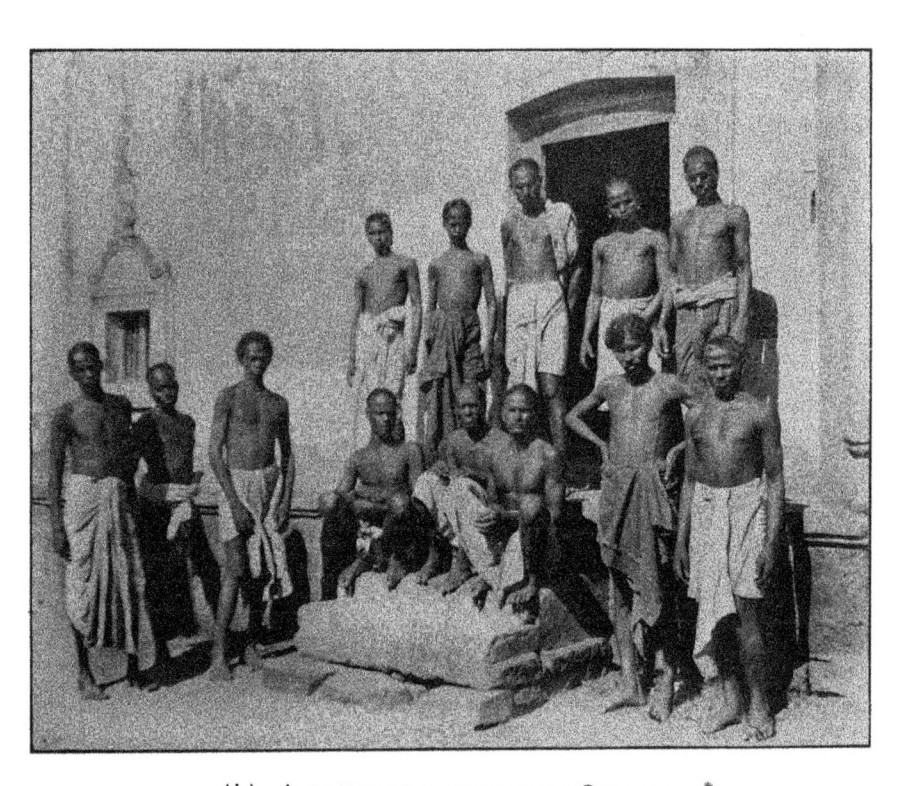

(*b.*) A GROUP OF BETTER CLASS OORIYAS.

The Nepalese also eats largely of the better-class cereals—wheat, maize, and good millets.

DIET VII.—NEPALESE CULTIVATORS (COOLIES OF POORER CLASSES).
Protein, 110 to 115 grms. Heat value, 3,000 to 3,200 calories.

Only a small percentage of the protein is derived from an animal source, usually 8 ounces of meat once or twice a week.

These dietaries, contrasted with those of the rice-eating Bengali, are very superior not only in the gross quantities of protein consumed, but also in the manner in which the total protein is made up. They serve to illustrate the general law, that where there is free choice of food, hard muscular labour demands a liberal supply, and insists, when financially possible, on a generous proportion of an animal protein in the daily dietary.

As might be expected, the dietaries of these hill-tribes permits of a high level of nitrogenous interchange. From the results of investigations the following conclusions were arrived at with regard to the degree of protein metabolism* obtained with different dietaries :

	Nitrogen Metabolized per Kilo of Body Weight.
Nepalese Bhutias	0·42 grm.
Tibetan and Bhutan	0·35 ,,
Sikhim Bhutias	0·25 ,,
Nepalese	0·18 to 0·25 grm.
Anglo-Indian and Eurasian students	0·196 grm.
Other Anglo-Indian and Eurasian students	0·203 ,,
Bengal students (residential Government hostel)	0·148 ,,
Bengali students (private messes)	0·116 ,,
Students and servants	0·111 to 0·115 grm.
Two Bengali assistants	0·137 grm.
Beharis	0·145 ,,

These results should be contrasted with those obtained on—

	Nitrogen per Kilo of Body Weight Daily.
Scientific workers (Chittenden)	
Members of the Medical Corps (Chittenden)	0·12 to 0·13 grm.
Athletes (Chittenden)	
Poorer classes in Japan (Oshima)	0·177 grm.
Average European (Voit)	0·270 ,,

The significance of these results on physique and the general well-being of the body will be discussed in another connection.

* Scientific Memoirs, Government of India, No. 37, p. 222 ; also Memoir, No. 34.

At present it will be sufficient to point out the close similarity that exists between the quantity Chittenden has found amply sufficient to meet all the protein needs of the body and the average level of nitrogenous interchange in Bengalis.

Study 6.—An inquiry was made into the dietaries of the aboriginal tribes of Chota Nagpur in Bengal. The facts obtained go far to corroborate the finding of Dr. Harry Campbell as to the mixed form of alimentation shown by those races who have not yet reached the stage of cibiculture.

Some of these tribes have begun to cultivate the ground and raise crops ; some, on the other hand, live on what they can obtain without agriculture. The more highly civilized and Hindüized, such as the Pators and Sawanis, do not eat cow, buffalo, or pig ; the Mundas and Uraons of Dravidian extraction eat all kinds of flesh, including rats, snakes, insects, jackals, pigs, lizards, etc. —in fact, anything they can catch.

The Pators and Sawanis eat all other kinds of flesh, except that forbidden by the Hindu religion, and are particularly fond of goat. The Sawanis do not possess any land to rear goats, so that they have developed into a caste of professional thieves, the principal thing stolen by them being goats, which they promptly eat.

As the Mundas practically never milk their cows, infants who lose their mothers have a very poor chance of surviving.

The Todas, a pastoral tribe in the Nilghiri Hills of Southern India, are of more than ordinary interest from a dietetic standpoint. They are totally unacquainted with vegetable food, and live entirely on milk and buffalo meat or other animals that they can capture. They know nothing of salt, and have no desire for it. In this respect they exhibit the same characteristics as carnivora elsewhere. It has been shown, indeed, to be a universal rule that in all times and in all lands those people who live entirely upon animal food either never have heard of salt, or, if they possess salt, avoid it ; whereas the people whose staple food is vegetable, have the greatest desire for salt, and regard it as an indispensable article of diet.* The Bushmen of South Africa live by the chase, and do not use salt. Similarly, the Kirghese live on meat and milk ; the Bedouins in Arabia live on meat ; the Indians of North America, hunters and fishermen ; the shepherds of the South American pampas, who live

* Bunge, " Physiological and Pathological Chemistry "

entirely on meat and regard vegetable food as fit only for animals —none of these make use of salt, although there is no scarcity of it in any of these places.

It will be evident, therefore, that the aboriginal tribes of Chota Nagpur live on a mixed diet, a large part of the protein constituent of which is derived from an animal source. Taking the average of the dietaries investigated, over half the protein is provided by the animal kingdom in one or other form. The following is a fair average of the food consumption:

Average Diet.	Approximate Value.	
	Proximate Principles.	Calories.
Rice .. .. .. 20 ozs. Dal .. .. .. 2 ,, Vegetables .. .. 6 ,, Meat .. .. .. 6 ,, Milk .. .. .. 4 ,,	Protein .. .. 80 grms. Carbohydrates .. 500 ,, Fat .. .. 50 ,,	2,800

Of the total protein about 35 grammes is derived from an animal source. It will be noticed that meat forms a much larger part of the dietary than is the case with the inhabitants of the plains of Bengal. On the other hand, there is a smaller quantity than that found to be present in the dietaries of the hill-tribes of Darjeeling.

Of the 80 to 85 grammes of protein, 60 grammes are absorbable, which would mean the metabolism of 0·17 grammes per kilo of body weight. This is a considerably higher level of nitrogenous interchange than the Bengali attains, and brings these aborigines up to about the standard of the poorest Nepalese.

Study 7.—A considerable amount of information was collected with regard to the food and dietaries of the fighting castes of the United Provinces and the Punjab. In these provinces rice is no longer the staple foodstuff, its place being taken to a large extent by wheat amongst the better-fed classes, and by maize and the different millets amongst the poorest classes. As might be expected, the dietaries of the good-fighting tribes are very superior to those of Behar or Lower Bengal. The superiority is largely due to the substitution of wheat and maize for rice. Good-class wheat contains up to almost twice as much protein as rice, and its protein shows a very much higher coefficient of absorbability. In the food consumption of the races from which the best material is obtained for the Indian Army, a considerable quantity of animal matter has a place. Milk and its various preparations form very important elements of the dietary with all classes.

As we shall have occasion to discuss the dietaries of these fighting tribes and the results seemingly obtained from them in another connection, it will be sufficient at present to give the food consumption of the Sikh—one of the most widely known of the fighting races of India.

1. As children. They, like most of the children of India, are breast-fed for a long period—about two and a half years. After the first year, or year and a half, the mother's milk is supplemented by fresh cow's milk diluted with an equal quantity of water. Towards the end of the period of suckling the child is given a morning feed of curdled milk—a sort of junket—4 ounces daily.

2. At two and a half years of age the child is weaned. He is then given four meals a day, the aggregate consisting of the following quantities of food materials, which represent the averages up to early adult life :

Approximate Value.

Milk	8 ozs.*	
Curd	2 ,, †	
Wheat	8 ,,	Protein, 50 to 60 grms.
Rice	4 ,,	Heat value, 2,000 to 2,250 calories.
Dal	2 ,,	
Sugar	2 ,,	
Vegetables	2 ,,	
Butter	1 oz.	

In addition, the child, at the age of three years, begins to take meat in small quantities, usually two or three times a month.

3. Young adults living in their villages are able to obtain large quantities of cow's milk and various kinds of animal food, such as goat's flesh, mutton, fowls (male fowls only), venison, bacon, eggs, ducks, pigeons, fish. The better off the family happens to be, the greater is the average amount of animal food in the dietary. Beef is never eaten, the cow being a sacred animal. The average dietary is as follows :

Approximate Value.

Milk	16 ozs.	
Wheat	24 ,,	
Butter	2 ,,	Protein, 125 to 130 grms.
Dal	3 ,,	Heat value, 3,750 to 4,000 calories.
Vegetables	6 ,,	
Meat	4 ,,	

* And upwards. † Morning.

Of the total protein, 35 to 45 per cent. is derived from an animal source. The large amount of milk in the dietaries of these people is very noticeable.

From the coefficients of protein absorption obtained for these foodstuffs in India, the level of protein metabolism may easily be calculated. Thus milk, butter, and meat provide 45 grammes protein, of which 43 grammes will be absorbed; and the cereals and vegetables provide 83 grammes, of which 75 per cent., or 62 grammes, will be absorbed. Therefore the total protein absorbed is 105 grammes, or 16·8 grammes nitrogen per man daily. The average weight of the Sikh is 68 kilos, which would mean a metabolism of 0·25 gramme of nitrogen per kilo of body weight. These are the minimum figures.

As will be evident, the diet of the Sikhs in their own homes is quite up to that of European standards. A minimum protein metabolism of 105 grammes daily, equal, in the case of the Sikh, to an interchange of 0·25 gramme of nitrogen per day, places him on an equal footing with the better-fed races of mankind, and very much superior to the rice-eating Bengali, and most of the other races of the plains of India.

It is of interest in this connection to examine the dietary of recruits on joining their regiment. The food and quantities per man are as follows:

		Approximate Value.
Milk	16 ozs.	
Butter	2¼ ,,	
Wheat	26 ,,	Protein, 135 grms.
Dal	3 ,,	Heat value, 4,000 calories.
Mutton	3 ,,	
Sugar	¼ oz.	
Vegetables	6 ozs.	

Besides this, recruits frequently purchase other delicacies out of their pay. About 40 grammes of the total protein is animal in nature, and the level of protein metabolism attained on the above diet works out at a daily interchange of 110 grammes, or 17·6 grammes of nitrogen per man daily. The above dietaries, which understate rather than overstate the case, are given in detail, as it is not uncommon to see such loose statements as the following made: "Hindus live entirely on rice." Sikhs are Hindus, therefore "Sikhs live on rice." "Sikhs live entirely on vegetable food." As a matter of fact, as will be seen when we come to examine the dietaries of the well-developed races of Northern India, the truth is that the foodstuffs made use of are of excellent quality, and sufficient in quantity to render them equal, if not superior, to the standard dietaries generally accepted in Europe and America. Further, it may be again insisted on that animal food in some form practically always enters into the composition of the dietaries of the great mass of the people. Milk is very cheap, except in the large towns, and, in its various preparations, forms an important element even in the food of the poorest. Ghi—butter that has been boiled and allowed to cool—is partaken of by all except those actually in absolute want.

Study 8.—As it is the custom in India for all mothers to suckle their offspring for at least the first year, it is of importance to know the composition of the Indian mother's milk. It would be very desirable if this could be obtained for the different tribes and races in India, and thus be able to determine if the difference in physique, stamina, etc., so evident amongst the several races, is accompanied by variations in the nutritive value of the infant's food. Such differences, other things being equal, would be expected—that is, a well-developed, well-fed mother would be more likely to be able to secrete milk of high nutritive value than a poorly developed, ill-fed woman. Owing to the many difficulties blocking the way, so far as we are aware, no statistics are available on this point. A certain number of analyses of the milk of Bengali women were made in the Physiological Department of the Calcutta Medical College with the following results :*

	Bengali Mother's Milk.	European Mother's Milk.
Protein	1·20 per cent.	1·6 per cent.
Carbohydrates	5·90 ,,	6·5 ,,
Fat	2·80 ,,	3·5 ,,
Minerals	0·24 ,,	0·2 ,,

Too much reliance cannot be placed on these differences in the several constituents, as it is well known how great the variations are in the composition of human milk from day to day, and even from hour to hour, even in the same woman. However, after making due allowance for this, it is evident that the milk secreted by Bengali women is considerably poorer in its different

* Dr. Lal Mohan Ghosal, " Food and Drugs," 1911.

elements than the milk of the average European women. It is also a well-recognized fact that the protein of human milk tends to decrease in amount as lactation proceeds, and that the milk of the mother does not get richer as the child grows older, but that the increasing demand for nutriment by the growing infant is met by supplying an increased quantity of milk.* It might, therefore, be expected that the lower composition of the Bengali mother's milk would be compensated for by the secretion of larger quantities. Such, however, is not the case.

The requirements of a healthy infant, as observed by Camerer and Feer, on an average is as follows :*

1st and 2nd months	..	..	600 grms. daily	..	20 ozs. daily.
2nd and 4th ,,	..	..	800 ,,	,, ..	27 ,, ,,
5th and 7th ,,	..	..	950 ,,	,, ..	32 ,, ,,
7th and 9th ,,	..	..	1,020 ,,	,, ..	34 ,, ,,
9th and 12th ,,	..	..	1,150 ,,	,, ..	39 ,, ,,

The average quantity of milk secreted by the European mother being calculated to be 1½ to 2 pints daily. In India, from observations on Bengali women, the daily quantity of milk secreted was found to be 1 to 1½ pints. The daily requirements of the infant were also tested by careful weightments of the child before and after each feeding, with the following results :

1st to 2nd months	..	..	400 grms. daily	..	14 ozs. daily.
2nd to 4th ,,	..	..	600 ,,	,, ..	20 ,, ,,
4th to 6th ,,	..	..	750 ,,	,, ..	27 ,, ,,
6th to 9th ,,	..	..	800 ,,	,, ..	28 ,, ,,
9th to 12th ,,	..	..	900 to 1,000 ,,	,,	30 to 35 ,, ,,

It would appear, therefore, so far as observations in India go, that the Bengali infant is not provided by Nature with as great a quantity of milk, nor with milk reaching the same high standard of chemical composition, as the European infant. This fact would appear to be a provision of Nature in providing a supply of food in accordance with the requirements of the infant. The average weight of the European newly born infant may be taken at 7·4 pounds, whereas the average Bengali new-born infant weighs 5·9 pounds at most.

The following table† shows the average weight of new-born infants of European and Indian mothers confined in the Eden Hospital, Calcutta :

* Hutchison, " Food and the Principles of Dietetics."
† Leicester, *Journal of Obstetrics and Gynæcology*, June, 1907.

Number of Confinements.	Average Weight of Infant.	Variations Observed.
87 Europeans	7·4 lbs.	Maximum, 10·56 lbs. Minimum, 5·56 ,,
142 natives	5·9 ,,	Maximum, 8·27 ,, Minimum, 4·09 ,,

By contrasting the quantities of nutritive materials available for a Bengali and European infant of six months of age, these differences are clearly brought out:

Proximate Principles.	European Infant.	Bengal Infant.
Protein	14 grms.	9·6 grms.
Carbohydrates	59 ,,	47·2 ,,
Fat	30 ,,	22·4 ,,

From careful observations on the influence of the mother's diet on the composition of her milk, it was found that fat is the only ingredient of the milk on which diet produces any effect. Baumm and Illner record a rise of 1 per cent. with a highly nitrogenous and with a very abundant mixed dietary; whereas an abundant supply of carbohydrates has no influence on the amount of fat, and an increased amount of fat eaten seems to diminish rather than increase the amount of cream in the milk. Observations on cows fed on a highly nitrogenous bean diet, which produces milk greater in quantity and richer in quality than any other diet, would afford strong evidence of the importance of the protein element in the diet of the mother in influencing the chemical composition of her milk.

The fact that the dietary of the Bengali is very poor in protein and fat, whilst comparatively rich in carbohydrates, in all probability is sufficient to account for the differences met with in the milk of the Bengali when contrasted with that of European women.

The importance of an adequate supply of nutritive materials in the food of the infant has never been called in question by even the most rabid advocates of the superior merits of a low protein dietary. It may therefore be accepted that the lower quantities of the several constituents available in the case of Bengali children will tend to be accompanied by a lesser body weight and a slower rate of growth. This state of affairs, acting continuously through countless generations, must eventually lead to the evolution of a race whose individuals are relatively on a lower scale of physical development than that of the better-fed races of European countries. If, after the period of suckling is over, Bengali children were given liberal quantities of the materials on which growth depends, they might be expected to make up the lost ground to some extent, although the general opinion of animal breeders is against such a contention, it being widely held amongst these classes that if a strong, well-developed animal of whatever species is wanted, it must be well fed from birth. As has been shown, however, the Bengali never receives sufficient protein at any age to do much more than meet the pressing requirements of ordinary wear and tear, so that the excess of protein available for the growth and building up of the nitrogenous tissues never reaches a high level.

In accordance with this chronic state of more or less nitrogenous starvation, we find the Bengali poor in physique, very poor in muscular tissue, the body fat at a minimum, and the average working man absolutely incapable of prolonged or sustained muscular efforts. The average body weight of the Bengali is 50 kilos, that of the European 65 to 70 kilos.

We may now turn from the consideration of the dietaries themselves to the study of the effects of those dietaries, particularly as regards their protein constituents.

CHAPTER V

THE PROTEIN REQUIREMENTS OF MANKIND

In an earlier chapter we examined the twofold function of food, and saw that it is essential for the growth and repair of the protoplasmic tissues, and necessary to furnish energy for the muscular and other work the body has to perform, and yield heat for the maintenance of the body temperature at a proper level.

Leaving aside for the present the question of mineral matters and water, the above requirements are met by the protein element on the one hand, and the total potential energy of the dietary on the other. Protein alone of the constituents of a diet is able to perform both functions; carbohydrates and fat are only capable of providing heat and potential energy. Dietaries may therefore be considered from the standpoint of the protein element and total energy or heat value. The nutritive values of the fats and carbohydrates are almost proportional to the amount of energy they can furnish; consequently, it is only important that the quantity of either, or both, be such that their total energy, when added to that of the protein of a diet, shall supply the total amount required by the body, due allowance being made for the decrease in the energy value, caused by the loss of a certain amount of the potential energy in the corresponding urine and fæces.*

In the present connection it is not necessary to discuss in detail the heat values of the dietaries examined, not because they are relatively of small importance, but for the reason that ordinarily the caloric value is quite sufficient to meet the demands of the body, if the diet is otherwise satisfactory. Further, as in the present volume, we are dealing more particularly with the light that may be thrown on the problems of nutrition from observations on the effects of tropical dietaries; the caloric

---

* Benedict, "The Nutritive Requirements of the Body."

value is not of such great importance as would be the case in European dietaries. The reason for this is that tropical food, being largely of a vegetable nature, any dietary that affords a sufficiency of the protein element is very unlikely to be deficient in carbonaceous material, but, indeed, will usually provide a potential energy considerably in excess of the ordinary dietary standard.

In connection with the work on dietaries in India, except where the potential energy is evidently of importance, we shall limit our consideration of the subject to the protein element.

There is just one aspect of carbon metabolism that we should like to refer to at once, as it has impressed itself very urgently on us whilst working with diets that provide a large fuel value, such as the gaol dietaries of Bengal. The usually accepted statements place the coefficient of carbohydrates absorption from different foodstuffs very high—as a rule, from 96 to 99 per cent. This result is arrived at by comparing the loss of carbohydrate, capable of being hydrolyzed into sugar, in the fæces with the total quantity presented in the diet. Now the Bengal gaol diets provide, in comparison with European standards, a very excessive amount of carbohydrates, sufficient in most cases to raise the energy metabolism to 60, or over 60, calories per kilo of body weight. Apparently the large quantities of carbohydrate matter necessary for this great heat value are practically all absorbed, as only a very small percentage could be recovered from the fæces.

On thinking over the question how this great potential energy is made use of by Bengali prisoners, we have experienced considerable difficulty in accepting the customary explanation that it leaves the body in the form of heat and mechanical work, or is retained as fat. The ordinary working Bengali is a particularly thin individual, decidedly wanting in body fat, and his desire for, or capabilities of, muscular exertion are less than in any other race with whom we have had to do. The large masses of carbohydrate cannot, therefore, be burnt off in providing energy for muscular exertion, neither can it be fixed and stored in the body as fat. The demands for fuel for the maintenance of body heat in a tropical country should not be anything like so great as in colder climates; and yet the accepted standard for Europeans is from 40 to 45 calories per kilo of body weight, whilst prisoners in Indian gaols are provided with 60 to 70 calories.

The extremely meagre clothing of the poorer classes may create a certain demand for easily oxidizable material in the up-keep of the body temperature, particularly during the cold weather.

The question, therefore, arises : Seeing that a European in a cold climate, doing an average amount of work, can live quite well with 40 calories per kilo of body weight, whilst the Bengali prisoner, in a hot climate, doing the very minimum of work, is provided with 60 to 70 calories per kilo of body weight, what becomes of the great potential energy of the dietaries ? How does he get rid of it ? How is it dissipated ?

The answer to this question would appear to be threefold. A part of the carbohydrate, varying in amount according to the needs of the body, is absorbed and made use of to supply the energy necessary for the maintenance of body heat and that essential for the work of the body ; a part undergoes little or no change in the bowel, and passes out undissolved. This is probably due to its being bound up with cellulose, so that the digestive juices are unable to penetrate to the starch granules and set up changes essential for absorption. A third part is broken up in the digestive tract by excessive micro-organismal fermentation, which, beginning in the stomach, is contained in the intestines. By this last method a very large percentage of the total potential energy of the diet may be dissipated through the conversion of its starch or sugar into carbon dioxide, methane, hydrogen, acetic acid, butyric acid, etc., and other fermentative products of low caloric value.

This loss, which may be considerable in amount depending upon the extent of intestinal fermentation, will tend to reduce the fuel value of the diet, and may afford a likely explanation of the remarkable want of body fat in the great majority of the working population of Bengal. So far as we know, there is no method by which this loss can even be approximately computed —at least, by chemical means ; but that it is an important factor in reducing the potential value of the food will be readily admitted when it is considered that even with gaol dietaries, which are exceedingly rich in carbohydrates, the storing of fat is practically nil, whilst in the working coolie of Bengal, living in a condition of more or less nitrogen starvation, neither body fat nor properly developed muscular tissues are usually to be found.

It is evident from the above considerations that the ordinary methods of determining the digestibility and absorption of the carbohydrates and fat of dietaries, may not give anything like accurate results.

This objection does not hold when dealing with protein. The fæcal nitrogen may be accepted as a true measure of the protein lost to the body, whatever may be the actual form in which it is excreted. Thus, in conditions of excessive putrefaction, the nitrogen may be largely represented as masses of bacteria. However, as nitrogen cannot be lost nor created in the bowel, any change of form will have no influence on the actual quantity present. One other point in this connection may be referred to —viz., the nitrogen eliminated in the fæces that really has been metabolized, but has been made use of in the formation of the intestinal juices. There is very little doubt that vegetable dietaries, such as those of India, require a very much greater secretion of the several digestive juices than the ordinary mixed dietary of Europeans, and that relatively there is a greater loss of metabolized nitrogen from this source than should be the case.

Strictly speaking, the nitrogen derived from the secretions of the bowel is not really loss from the protein intake of the food, but in actual effect it comes to exactly the same thing. Whether the fæcal nitrogen is derived from the protein of the food or from the intestinal secretions, it is lost so far as the body is concerned. If a diet requires great quantities of the intestinal juices for its digestion, a corresponding great increase in the fæcal nitrogen from this source will be determined, and a corresponding amount of nitrogen will be withdrawn from the body to provide the materials necessary for the digestive secretions. We have, therefore, in the determination of the fæcal nitrogen a true measure of the total waste of protein corresponding to the dietary for the period during which the investigation is being carried out. With a knowledge of the protein intake during that period the co-efficient of protein absorption from the food can easily be arrived at.

Having decided that dietaries may be considered from the view-point of their total protein and energy values, and that the potential energy is usually sufficient, if not excessive, the only question we are directly concerned with at present is the protein element.

The Protein Requirements of the Body.

The problem presented in determining the daily requirements of the body for protein is one concerning which there has been a good deal of controversy, and one to which, up to the present, no definite solution has been furnished. Several different methods of attacking this problem have been devised.

Thus it has been shown that, on an average, all over the world where a sufficiency of food is available, mankind consumes at least 100 grammes of protein daily. The Japanese and Hindus have been regarded as notable exceptions; but on closer examination such will not be found to be the case. Both Japanese and Hindus make use of large, rather than small, quantities of protein where a free choice of food can be afforded. Further, as has been exemplified by the dietaries of the jinricksha men of Japan, and hill-tribes of Bengal, and amongst the better-fed classes of the plains of India, it is not simply a matter of increasing the quantities of the ordinary foodstuffs consumed—this, indeed, does take place to some extent—but, what is more noticeable and of greater importance, is that there is a demand for foods that are of a highly nitrogenous nature. The increasing amounts of protein taken by different individuals when the severity and amount of work which they are called upon to do increases, v. Noorden explains very simply by an increase in the amount of the ordinary food, as made use of when the work performed is not of a severe nature. This naturally increases the protein intake.* Whilst this may be the case in dealing with dietaries in which the protein element is present in quantities reaching the European standards, the evidence afforded by those engaged in hard muscular work on dietaries of the type common to the tropics, would show that an increase of their highly carbonaceous food materials is not sufficient to meet the requirements of the body; but that highly nitrogenous foods, if possible of an animal nature, are demanded for the maintenance of the musculature and power of doing work. The large additions made to the otherwise carbonaceous dietaries of the jinricksha men of Japan and dandy carriers of India in the form of animal protein afford a considerable weight of evidence on this point.

The almost universal desire of mankind for a dietary contain-

* V. Noorden, " The Physiology of Metabolism," p. 305.

ing at least 100 grammes of protein daily, despite variations in race, country, climate, and dietetic habits, is very significant, and has been acknowledged by most observers as conclusive evidence of the need of at least this amount of protein. This argument is all the more forcible and convincing in view of the fact that all the world over protein, particularly animal protein, is one of the most expensive constituents of the food, often involving a good deal of labour and sacrifice to procure.

On the data furnished by freely chosen diets in different parts of the world have been founded the standard dietaries which have been given in detail in a former chapter. The most popular and widely accepted of these is, perhaps, that laid down by Voit, which provides 118 grammes of assimilable protein for an energetic man doing a moderate amount of work. Up to comparatively recent times the approximate correctness of these standards has never been called in question. They were regarded as the minimal quantities that should enter into any well-balanced diet, but not as bounds beyond which it was dangerous to exceed.

It has been objected to these standards, based on the dietetic customs and habits of mankind, that, although the consumption of over 100 grammes of protein daily is almost universal, it does not necessarily follow that it is to the welfare of the body. It has been pointed out that " habits and cravings are certainly very unreliable indices of true physiological requirements ;" that " dietetic requirements and standard dietaries are not to be founded upon the so-called cravings of appetite and the instinctive demands for food, but upon reason and intelligence, reinforced by definite knowledge of the real necessities of the bodily machinery." Chittenden even goes so far as to say : " Standards which have been adopted more or less generally throughout the civilized world, based primarily on the assumption that man instinctively and independently selects a diet which is best adopted to his individual needs, are open to grave suspicion. The true food requirements of the body, under any conditions, cannot be ascertained with any degree of accuracy by observations of what people are in the habit of eating." Mankind, according to Chittenden, is guided by blind instinct or the leadings of a capricious appetite, and eats as much of the higher and more expensive protein food materials as he can afford. Certainly, the only people who fail to attain the ordinary protein standard are those who are too poor to afford the cost of the average diet; or who, living on a very bulky vegetable diet, are unable to consume sufficient of their foodstuffs to provide the amount of assimilable protein present in Voit's standard.

There is little doubt, therefore, that the evidence of mankind points indisputably to a desire for protein up to European standards. As soon as a race can provide itself with such amounts, it promptly does so; as soon as financial considerations are surmounted, so soon the so-called "vegetarian Japanese" or Hindu raises his protein intake to reach the ordinary standard of mankind in general.

With regard to the objections raised by Chittenden as to the fundamental importance of the dietetic habits of mankind being taken into consideration in determining the protein requirements, all that need be said is that he appears to stand practically alone in upholding this view. "It is an initial objection to Chittenden's view, which is not easily met, that it contravenes all human experience. If he is right, then all the world up to this time, with the exception, perhaps, of a few faddists, has been wrong. Gluttony has somehow become universal. It is 'Chittenden contra mundum.'"* "It is inconceivable that all mankind, under the most diverse conditions, should have fallen into the same mistake. Such a unanimity means no mistake, but a physiological discovery. Natural instinct or primitive experience has guided the different varieties of our species in their selection of viands suitable to their geographical situation and modes of life, has restrained them within proper bounds in their consumption of these, and has taught them to combine and balance the different constituents of these in a way on which chemical science can scarcely improve."*

Hutchison, in discussing the relative weight to be attached to instinct and to greed respectively, in determining the dietetic habits of mankind, says that there is at least strong *a priori* reason for the belief that, in matters of diet, what has been adopted *semper et ubique et ab omnibus* is fundamentally right.

Sir William Roberts says: "The generalized food customs of mankind are not to be viewed as random practices adopted to please the palate or gratify an idle or a vicious appetite. These customs must be regarded as the outcome of profound instincts which correspond to certain wants of the human economy.

* Sir James Crichton-Browne, "Parsimony in Nutrition."

They are the fruit of a colossal experience accumulated by countless millions of men through successive generations . . . and are fitted to yield to observation and study lessons of the highest scientific and practical value."

Another method that has been put forward as a means of determining the actual needs of the body for protein is that based on Folin's observations on the constancy, under varying conditions, of the output of creatinine and neutral sulphur in the urine. Folin's work and the deductions therefrom have already been discussed at considerable length in the introductory chapter; it will not, therefore, be necessary to refer to them in detail in the present connection. It is generally acknowledged that protein is only really essential to keep in repair the nitrogenous tissues of the body, and that its function of supplying heat can be equally well undertaken by fats and carbohydrates. It would therefore appear probable that, if the heat value of a dietary were satisfactory owing to the presence of a sufficiency of these two constituents, the amount of protein necessary would only be that required to cover the loss from tissue wear and tear. With the advent of a reliable method of estimating the katabolism of protein involved in the disintegration of the true tissues, the problem of the nitrogenous requirements of the body from this standpoint would appear to be solved. Such a method has been supposed to be forthcoming in the determination of the creatinine-nitrogen of the urine, which has been regarded as a measure of the endogenous or tissue metabolism.

If the nitrogen in the form of creatinine were a measure of the katabolism of the tissue cells, then the heat value of a diet being sufficient, the same amount of nitrogen supplied in the food as lost to the body in the form of creatinine should be sufficient to meet the protein requirements of the body, make good the loss due to true tissue change, and maintain the subject in a condition of nitrogenous equilibrium.

The average amount of this creatinine-nitrogen is 0·6 gramme daily, remaining, according to Folin, practically constant, whether the diet be protein-rich or protein-free. The rational deduction to be drawn from this argument would be, if the creatinine-nitrogen is any measure of the protein requirements of the body, that under the stated conditions 0·6 gramme of assimilated nitrogen should be sufficient to maintain the body in nitrogenous equilibrium and insure the integrity of the tissue cells.

The fact that approximately ten times this amount of nitrogen is necessary in a dietary in order to maintain the body in nitrogenous equilibrium, when the caloric value of the diet is sufficient, would show that Folin's deductions regarding the creatinine-nitrogen as a measure of endogenous metabolism do not cover the facts, or, if it be such a measure, then there must be a large demand for protein in the body beyond that required to repair tissue waste and make good its loss.

From an analysis of the more recent work on creatinine excretion, we have shown in our introduction that the small and constant quantity eliminated daily cannot be made use of as evidence to support the arguments of those who consider that the protein requirements of the body would be covered by the presence of a very limited amount of nitrogen in the daily food.

It is just possible that creatinine is a partial measure of the nitrogenous interchanges going on within muscular tissue, and that 0·6 gramme of creatinine-nitrogen represents to some extent the degree of this special type of metabolism. This would leave out of consideration the interchanges taking place between the cells of all other tissues and the lymph, and the large supply of fluid protein not actually incorporated into the material of the living cell—the " labile protein " of physiologists.

In the light of recent researches on the constitution of the protein molecule and on the demands of the tissues, not for nitrogen merely, but for nitrogen in certain combinations, or complexes of molecules, it is possible that, in the providing of even 0·6 gramme of nitrogen in the form required by the muscle cells, large quantities of protein taken in the food will require to be broken down into their different units in order that the suitable " building-stones " may be available in sufficient amount. However, without an accurate knowledge of the total nitrogenous requirements, and lacking any reliable method of determining them, these possibilities are merely interesting speculations. The fact that in the case of the fasting subject the excretion of nitrogen is far in excess of the amount which, according to Folin, corresponds to disintegrated tissue protein, would show clearly that his deductions regarding the significance of creatinine in the urine as a measure of the protein requirements of the tissues cannot be correct.

An attempt has been made to arrive at the true protein requirements of man by studying the conditions that obtain during starvation. It was thought that in the amount of nitrogen excreted during fasting experiments there would be obtained a measure of the quantity of protein necessary to make good the loss from tissue disintegration. However, it is found that excretion of nitrogen during hunger or fasting is modified by a variety of circumstances, particularly the amount of "labile" or circulating proteins and the condition of the body with regard to presence of fat.

For the first few days after the withdrawal of food the excretion of nitrogen is directly dependent upon the protein intake and decomposition during the preceding days. The amount of labile protein present in the body varies with the level of protein metabolism during the period immediately before the fast commenced. If this level beforehand is high, the nitrogen output during the first few days is large; and if low, the output is correspondingly small.

According to Voit, about 8 per cent. of the stable protein and 70 per cent. of the labile protein of the organism are decomposed during starvation, the latter being completely used up within three days. From the fourth and fifth day onwards only stable tissue protein remains for oxidation, the labile having disappeared. Similarly with regard to the glycogen stored in the body, which can act as a protein sparer. It is practically exhausted by the third day of fasting, and, as a result, the protein metabolism, as measured by the nitrogen excretion, shows a temporary rise. After some initial variations, the nitrogenous katabolism in man gradually decreases during the course of starvation. In the first ten days the nitrogen excretion seldom falls below 10 grammes, but later on falls still lower.*

An average of the results obtained from different fasting experiments shows that the nitrogen excreted in the urine from the fifth day of starvation onwards is about 5 grammes per day. This amount is, however, not sufficient to supply the energy required by the body.

It is estimated that only about 10 per cent. of the total energy is derived from tissue disintegration, the remaining 90 per cent. being supplied by the large store of fat present in the body when in an ordinary condition of nutrition. So long as this store of fat lasts the protein tissues will be drawn on mainly to meet the

* v. Noorden, " Physiology of Metabolism."

demands of the organism for nitrogen. When the store of fat gives out, there will be an increase in the amount of tissue breakdown, since now all forms of energy will come from the katabolism of protein, and this will be accompanied by a marked increase in the output of nitrogen—"the pre-mortal rise in the nitrogen excretion."

Accepting the figure 5 grammes as representing the urinary nitrogen, and allowing 0·5 gramme nitrogen for other modes of excretion, the conclusion may be arrived at that the minimum amount of assimilated nitrogen necessary to prevent the disintegration of tissue proteins is 5·5 grammes.

If this amount be given to a starving man, it will be found that it is by no means sufficient to establish nitrogenous equilibrium and prevent tissue breakdown. The smallest amount of nitrogen in the food on which it is possible to establish nitrogenous equilibrium is some three to four times the amount excreted during starvation. If the fasting man, however, has a large store of fat, or, if large quantities of fats and carbohydrates are taken as food, the sparing action of these materials may be sufficiently great to allow of nitrogenous metabolism being maintained on quantities as small as 5 or 6 grammes of nitrogen per day—*i.e.*, "Man can keep the protein store of his organism unaltered in amount on a supply of protein which lies far below the amount decomposed during starvation."

This figure may therefore be accepted as representing the lower limits of nitrogenous metabolism, and further decrease of assimilable protein in the food, no matter how abundant the carbonaceous element may be, will entail a falling back of the organism on its own nitrogenous tissues. Numerous observations and experiments by Chittenden, Neumann, Sivén, Klemperer, Peschal, and others, have shown that nitrogenous equilibrium can be maintained with a diet containing about 6 grammes of nitrogen, even when the total energy value was not excessive. In Chittenden's experiments the potential energy was below the ordinary accepted standards. As will be evident, also, the inhabitants of Bengal corroborate this finding on a large scale and over long periods of time.

For the present we may leave this point, accepting the finding that the metabolism of about 6 grammes of nitrogen is the physiological minimum on which mankind is able to make good the wear and tear of his protoplasmic tissues when the demands of the body for energy are fully met by an abundant supply of carbohydrates and fats. This amount may be regarded as the minimum quantity of protein essential for existence, and must be carefully distinguished from the quantity necessary to maintain the body in the highest degree of efficiency.

By none of the methods discussed above can a definite answer be given to the question, What are the protein requirements of the body ? The fact that the body is ever striving to adapt the protein decomposition to the intake, and that it can establish itself in a condition of nitrogenous equilibrium on very varying quantities of protein, is the great cause of the difficulties that beset the path of those engaged in finding a conclusive reply to the above question. This power of the organism of being able to maintain itself in nitrogenous equilibrium on the most diverse amounts of protein could only mean that sooner or later controversy must arise as to what particular level of interchange is best for the efficiency, economy, and welfare of the body. The question, therefore, instead of being, What are the protein needs of the body ? becomes, What level of protein metabolism is most advantageous ?

As has been demonstrated at considerable length, it is the universal opinion of those most interested in furnishing a correct answer—viz., mankind in general—that at least 100 grammes of protein daily is necessary if the body is to be maintained in a condition of health and efficient for the average degree of labour it is called on to perform ; that the protein requirement is influenced by work, hard labour demanding sooner or later an increase in the protein constituent of the diet. Accepting for the moment the recognized view that the energy of muscular work comes from the carbonaceous and not from the nitrogenous constituents of the body, the fact remains that increased labour creates a demand for protein food. This demand is all the more noticeable the poorer the ordinary foodstuffs are in their protein content. In an ordinary mixed dietary this desire for protein is met by an increase in the total amount of food consumed ; but in tropical dietaries, which are usually highly carbonaceous, and not infrequently bulky, a highly nitrogenous food is taken in addition, or replaces some of the more carbonaceous materials. This point is well exemplified by the great consumption of animal food amongst those who do really hard labour in India and Japan. With the mixed dietaries of Europe and America the desire for increased protein during hard labour is obscured, or at least is explained away as a mere incident of the necessary corresponding increase of food.

Physiological opinion with regard to the rôle of protein as a source of energy for muscular contraction has begun to swing back to some extent from the extreme views originally held. Thus Liebig believed that protein was the only food capable of supplying the energy of muscular contraction. When this was proved not to be the case, opinion veered round to the other extreme, and carbonaceous matter was regarded as the only source. At the present time it is considered most likely that muscular contraction makes no special demand on one nutritive constituent of the food more than another, all being made use of for the supply of the necessary potential energy. When the deduction is made that only comparatively small quantities of nitrogen are necessary because the body is able, seemingly, to burn up all the protein that is given to it within twenty-four hours; when, similarly, the fact that the urinary nitrogen is not found to be greatly increased during muscular excretion is taken to mean that protein is of little or no importance as a source of the energy of muscular contraction, we are going beyond the facts, and beyond what is warranted in the present state of our knowledge. All that is certain is that, on the average, quantities of nitrogen and sulphur, corresponding closely with the quantities of those materials absorbed from the food, are excreted within that period. The changes that may have taken place in protein from the time it is broken down into the hydrolyzed products of digestion until it eventually appears in the urine as nitrogen are absolutely unknown. It certainly appears somewhat rash to jump to the conclusion that the great proportion of the protein of a standard diet is of no real service to the organism, simply because the decomposition of protein keeps pace with the intake, and that seemingly the nitrogen absorbed from the food is rapidly eliminated.

That protein must be taken into consideration as a source of the energy of muscular work, leaving aside entirely its influence on the efficiency and well-being of the body as a machine, which influence cannot be measured and expressed in terms of so much excreted nitrogenous waste-products, Paton's investigations would make most probable. He found that the excretion of nitrogen was increased both during and after the performance

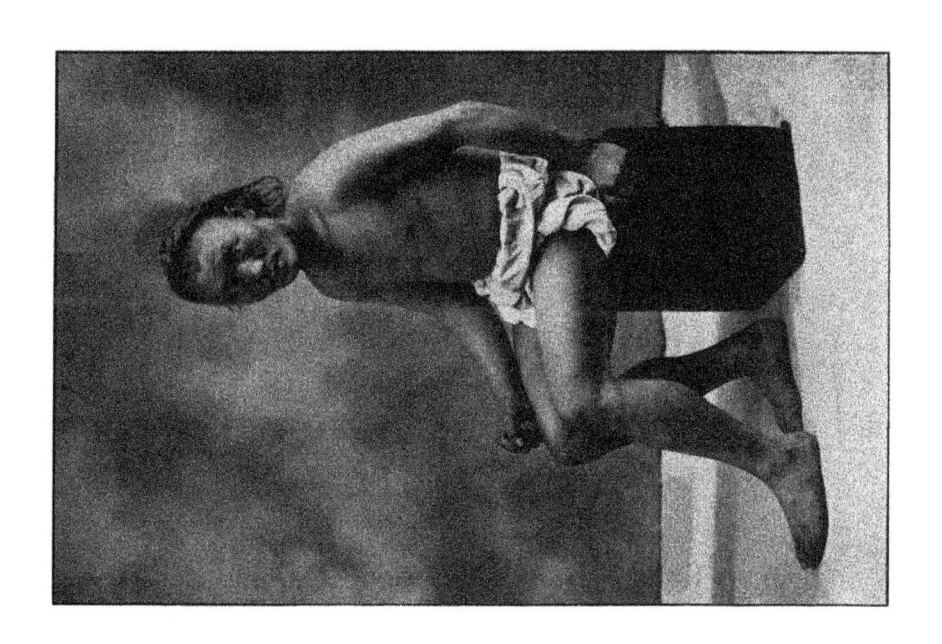

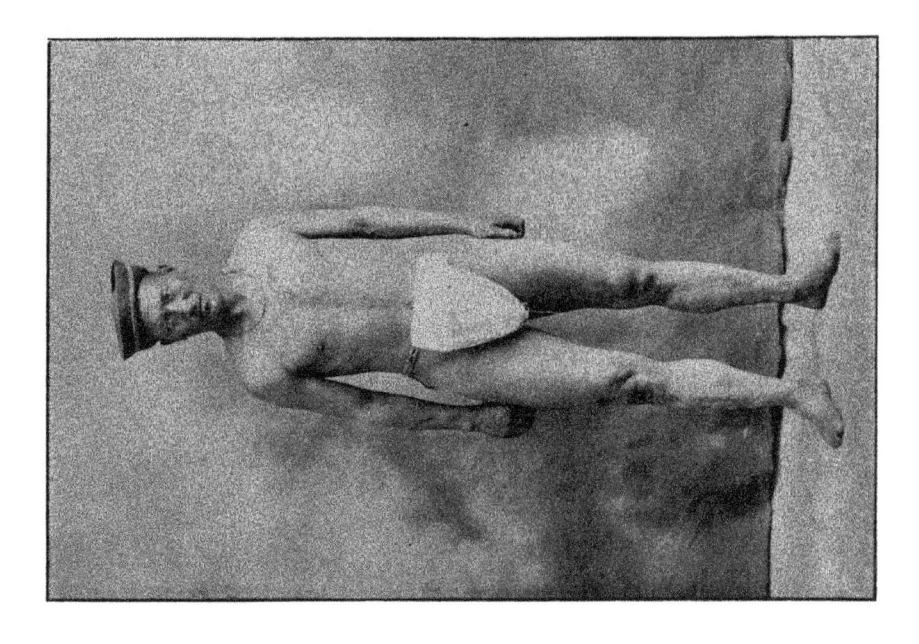

of work, and the metabolism of protein indicated by the increased nitrogen excretion amounted to 35 per cent. of the work done. The conclusion arrived at is that " when the body contains no stored protein, muscular exertion increases the output of nitrogen 15 per cent.; but if the body is in good condition "—that is, containing a store of circulating proteins—" the output of nitrogen is larger, because such proteins are consumed as a source of heat and energy; but the muscle fibres are not broken down in a greater proportion by the work they perform."*

Even if the excretion of nitrogen were entirely unaffected by work, this would be no proof that none of the energy of muscular contraction comes from proteins. The excretion of nitrogen would be unaltered when proteins are oxidized within the body, whether in the one case their energy appeared in the form of heat, or in the other case it became diverted to muscular contraction.

In connection with this conception it is probable that in the work of the body generally, and in the work of muscle in particular, protein may be made use of according to the richness and liberality of the supply; in fact, it is known beyond doubt that the organism is prodigal of its protein when there is an abundance offered in the food, and most economical when the opposite conditions obtain. It can easily be imagined that with a free supply of protein the interchanges taking place in the nitrogenous tissues are ranged at a high level, the old building-stones are rapidly got rid of, and their place occupied by others manufactured from the amino-acids of digestion. This would not mean any increase in the excretion of nitrogen beyond that which would be the case on the theory that a very large proportion of the protein is short-circuited through the liver, changed into urea, and rapidly eliminated.

In the opposite condition, when the supply of protein is eventually cut off, or greatly diminished, the tissue cells, instead of eliminating their old or damaged building-stones, make use of them in the best manner possible to repair the waste essential to body work and growth, and even cut down the protein interchanges to the lowest possible level. This would mean that, although during muscular exertion there may be no great increase in the excretion of nitrogen, the tissue cells, on the other hand,

* Tibbles, "The Protein Requirement," *British Medical Journal*, vol. ii., 1911.

cannot be maintained at anything like the same high level of nutrition as when the supply of protein is liberal. That this view is correct would appear probable from the results of observations on the effects of establishing an animal on the lower limits of nitrogenous equilibrium—the carbonaceous constituents of the diet being abundant—and then causing an increase in the work performed. The animal will soon pass from its condition of nitrogen balance, and rapidly lose weight from the disintegration of its own tissues. In this experiment the heat value of the diet may be exceedingly abundant, and yet the extra work determines a disintegration of protein that cannot be met by the amount present in the food, nor by the makeshift arrangement of using over again the damaged building materials of the tissue cells. In this way the increasing demands of the body for protein during severe muscular exertion can be explained, and the importance of a high level of nitrogenous interchange in maintaining the tissues of the body in an efficient and economical condition can be understood. Until more is known concerning the changes that go on within the body from the digestion of protein until its elimination, it is impossible to say how much, or in what way, nitrogen is made use of in the work of muscle or in the other nitrogenous tissues.

As Stewart has pointed out in connection with the fate of protein within the body: "The fact that very soon after the introduction of proteins (as well as other food substances) into the blood the increased metabolism of them begins, is not of itself sufficient to show that they are destroyed without being built up into the protoplasm. For the protoplasm may have the power of rapidly assimilating the protein in the presence of an abundant supply, and of rapidly breaking down at the same time."*

It may be concluded, therefore, that so far as evidence afforded by the dietaries of mankind assists in determining the most advantageous level of protein metabolism, it points to at least 100 grammes of protein daily as the limit below which, on the average, nitrogenous interchange should not fall; that when hard muscular labour is performed, amounts considerably in excess of this are necessary; that the carbonaceous material of a dietary being sufficient, the fact that a larger amount of protein is required to maintain the body in nitrogenous equilibrium

* Stewart, "A Manual of Physiology," p. 470.

when at work than when resting, points indisputably to the importance of protein as a factor in the provision of energy for muscular contraction. The investigations of Paton, Stockman, Frentzel, and others afford further evidence of the important part played by protein in muscular work, and show that severe and excessive exercise is accompanied and followed by an increased elimination of nitrogen in the urine.

Further, we have attempted to demonstrate that, when an abundant supply of protein is available, the tissues, and particularly the muscular tissues, are in a position to replace disintegrated tissue with new material derived from the products of tryptic digestion—an opportunity not afforded them when the level of nitrogenous metabolism is low, in which case it is not improbable that the tissue cells have to make use of their old or damaged building-stones until such time as fresh material is forthcoming. It is not difficult to imagine that under such conditions the efficiency and economical working of the body may suffer, as compared with the more advantageous position which obtains when the protein metabolism is pitched at a high level; and this condition would be all the more marked and exaggerated when, in combination with a low level of nitrogenous metabolism, a high standard of functional activity is demanded, as in severe muscular exercises. Lastly, we have referred to the view that only a few grammes of nitrogen daily is needed, as the speedy elimination of the nitrogen taken as food is suggested to mean that the great proportion of it never reaches the tissues, being split off as ammonia, changed into urea in the liver, and rapidly excreted in the urine. While this, in all probability, does take place to a certain extent, it is by no means proved to occur with the greater part of the protein, and the weight of available evidence would locate the metabolism of proteins, as well as other food substances, within the tissue cells. It would appear much more probable that the bioplasm possesses the power of rapidly assimilating the products of tryptic digestion in the presence of an abundant supply, and thus being able to replace at once any worn, damaged, or fatigued elements, in this way maintaining the whole mass of the protoplasmic tissues at a high level of nutrition and efficiency. Considering the weight of the total nitrogenous tissues of an average man, and making allowance for a certain proportion of nitrogen probably made use of in the form of ammonia to maintain the intracellular alkalinity of the liver and other tissues, the metabolism of 100 grammes of protein, or 16 grammes of nitrogen, daily would not mean any excessive degree of tissue disintegration and rebuilding.

In round numbers it would entail an interchange of about 1 gramme of protein in every 150 grammes of protoplasm present in the body of the average man.

Reference has been made to the evidence afforded by the work of Folin, Chittenden, and others, and to the conditions that obtain during under-feeding and starvation. From the results obtained it has been shown that the physiological minimum of nitrogen interchange is reached when the absorption and assimilation is decreased to about 6 grammes daily, the heat value of the diet being large and almost entirely derived from carbohydrates and fat. Folin's investigations, on the other hand, would appear to show that endogenous or tissue metabolism of the body is a very trivial affair, requiring, if the creatinine-nitrogen of the urine is any index, an interchange of less than 1 gramme of nitrogen between the tissue cells and lymph. The general effect of these observations would be to show that the average quantity of protein consumed by mankind in his daily fare is far in excess of the true requirements of the body. We have dealt with some of the arguments that have been relied on, and discussed their bearing on the point at issue. The real question to be decided is : Can the body maintain itself in an efficient condition, as regards its physical development, capacity for work, and resistance to disease, in as satisfactory a manner on just that quantity of protein that has been shown experimentally to be sufficient, to establish nitrogenous equilibrium at its lowest level, or, are larger quantities of protein, and a higher plane of nutritive changes essential ?

The question is narrowed down to this : Accepting the view that the energy of muscular contraction can be and is to a considerable extent supplied by non-nitrogenous foodstuffs and the carbohydrate moiety of the protein molecule, are we, therefore, justified in advocating a large decrease in the protein intake as compared with the amount arrived at in standard dietaries ?

Is the amount of protein necessary for the repair of true tissue waste—Folin's endogenous metabolism—and that necessary to cover the loss from external secretions, hairs, epithelial scales, etc., all that is required by the system? If so, then a few grammes of protein daily is all that is absolutely essential. In other words, are we justified in believing that a diet should contain only the minimum amount of protein on which nitrogenous equilibrium can be established? If we are not justified in this belief, and admit that an extra quantity above this minimum is for the welfare of the body, then where is the line to be drawn? The question at once arises, if a small extra amount of protein beyond actual requirements, Rubner's margin of safety, is to the advantage of the protein-containing tissues, will a larger quantity—an increased margin of safety—not be to their still greater advantage?

The answer to these inquiries can only be sought in metabolism experiments and dietary studies not undertaken with a view of showing the possibility of man subsisting and doing a certain amount of work on a protein intake of one-third to one-half that of Voit's standard, but carried out on a large scale, under varying conditions, and over long periods of time, with the object of determining the effects of a low protein dietary on man's bodily and mental efficiency, susceptibility to disease, and general well-being.

To a consideration of the evidence that has, and is being, accumulated on this important problem we shall now turn. Chittenden's views and the opinions of those who uphold the merits of diets poor in protein are too well known to require detailed exposition; only a short synopsis, therefore, will now be given of the work that has been done from this standpoint, reserving for the following chapters its consideration and an account of the results obtained by later observers.

EXPERIMENTAL RESULTS OBTAINED WITH MAN AS REGARDS THE EFFECTS OF DIETS POOR IN PROTEIN.

There are a large number of scattered observations throughout the literature of metabolism dealing with the lower limits of protein intake. In the earlier experiments, when the protein intake was small in amount, the fuel value of the diet was high, and it was found that a large supply of non-nitrogenous food materials allows the organism to accommodate itself easily to a low protein dietary. Sivén[*] was the first to reduce the energy value of the diet to moderate proportions even when the protein

[*] V. Noorden, " Physiology of Metabolism," p. 300.

intake was exceedingly low. Chittenden, experimenting on himself, was able to maintain himself in nitrogenous equilibrium on 37 to 40 grammes protein, and 1,539 to 1,613 gross calories (= 0·64 to 0·70 grammes protein, and 27 to 28 calories per kilo of body weight).

The following table from v. Noorden* summarizes a few of these observations :

Authors.	Duration of Experiment.	Calories per Kilo of Weight.	Protein of Food.	Protein per Kilo of Weight.
	Days.		Grms.	Grms.
Klemperer	8	80	33	0·50
Caspari	5	66	49	0·71
Peschel	8	50	43	0·58
Hirschfeld	8	47	46	0·60
Sivén	6	42	39	0·66
Neumann	13	40	76	1·10
Chittenden	{ 6	28	40	0·70
	{ 6	27	37	0·64

In practically all these experiments the conditions were artificial, and do not correspond to those of everyday life. They were only carried out over short periods, so that it might reasonably be argued that the results would not hold good for long periods and under natural conditions.

It was reserved for Chittenden, as v. Noorden expresses it, " to replace such laboratory experiments by a truly physiological one on a large scale, and to furnish complete evidence in favour of the view that a low protein intake is not only sufficient, but efficient, for the bodily requirements."

Chittenden himself has been cited as " a monument of fidelity " to his own views, and is certainly very greatly endowed with the courage of his convictions. For over seven years he has subsisted on a diet remarkable for its low level of protein intake, and as yet without suggestion of anything but benefit to his health and efficiency. He maintains that his health, general physical condition, and mental power, have all alike benefited by the change to a diet poor in nitrogen. This experiment is absolutely unique, as accurate observations have been made at intervals during this long period of years to determine any signs of inadequacy, or any ill-effects on the health, strength, and capacity for work. Indeed, Chittenden is disposed to think

* v. Noorden, "Physiology of Metabolism," p. 300.

that he has done more work and led a more active life in every way during the period of this experiment, and with greater comfort and less fatigue than usual.

Two points of very great interest are brought out in the records of these observations: one was the very complete utilization of the daily food—the loss of nitrogen to the body per day through the fæces amounted to only 0·79 gramme on a mixed diet, containing a considerable quantity of matter not specially concentrated; the other is that this establishment of nitrogen equilibrium on a low protein intake was accomplished without increase in the daily intake of non-nitrogenous foods. During the periods of six days, when the nitrogen balance was investigated, the average heat value of the food per day was only a little over 1,600 calories.

Taking the data recorded, with an average body weight of 57 kilos, and with an average daily elimination of nitrogen for nearly nine months of 5·7 grammes, it is evident the nitrogen metabolized per kilo of body weight was exactly 0·1 gramme.

This is certainly a most remarkable result, even when the facts that Chittenden's body weight is well below the average, and that his activity was mental rather than physical, are taken into account. Different partial explanations have been advanced which would show that the experiment was carried out under the most favourable conditions for a minimum intake of protein, and for a low potential energy of the dietary. But no mental suggestion nor simplicity in the routine of life will explain how an average man carries on the ordinary duties of a professional worker for a period of seven years, according to Chittenden's latest statement, on a diet whose fuel value is only 1,600 calories, or 28 calories per kilo of body weight, unless the average amount hitherto considered absolutely necessary—viz., about 40 calories per kilo of body weight—is far above the true requirements. There are only two other possible explanations: either there is some fallacy in the figures giving the data during the two periods of six days each when a nitrogen balance was struck, so that they do not accurately represent the conditions that obtained during the whole period of observation, or, if the results obtained from this experiment are to be extended to mankind in general, the law of the conservation of energy as applied to human beings must be seriously called in question.

In this connection may be pointed out the surprisingly small quantities of food consumed by Chittenden during the days of the nitrogen balance. The dietaries are recorded in weights for cooked food, but the weight in the dry condition could not have reached more than 12 to 14 ounces daily, of which a very large proportion consisted of potatoes and lettuce-orange salad. With so large a quantity of vegetable material entering into the diet during the days of observation, it is all the more noticeable how very small the loss of nitrogen in the fæces proved to be. The very small quantities of food taken during the days of observation may be partly accounted for by the subject unconsciously living more abstemiously than usual, or perhaps choosing foodstuffs deficient in both protein and potential energy. That this explanation is not improbable is brought out in the following summary of the diet for June 23, 1904 :*

		Nitrogen Value.
Total weight of cooked diet, excluding fluids drunk ..	854 grms.	6·622 grms.
Weight of potatoes, strawberries, and lettuce-orange salad	445 ,,	0·957 ,,

That is, over half the gross weight of the cooked ration is made up of vegetable material which, as a matter of fact, is largely water, and which only offers one-seventh part of the total nitrogen of the diet. The potential energy of these materials is similarly deficient. By the choice of such foods, whilst there may be the feeling of satisfaction after a meal, the nitrogen and energy value can be brought to a very low level. It is quite possible, as Benedict[†] has shown in the case of a subject living on about 1,600 calories, that the body was not in energy equilibrium, but that there was an oxidation of the body fat with a retention of water, the body weight thus remaining fairly constant.

Chittenden experimented with three groups of subjects : the first consisted of professional men doing a minimum amount of muscular work ; the second was composed of volunteers from the Army Hospital Corps who took a moderate amount of exercise ; while the third group was made up of students engaged in active athletics. The study by Chittenden on himself referred to above is by far the most remarkable of those carried out on professional men.

The studies with thirteen soldiers from the Hospital Corps gave results very similar to those obtained with the professional men of the first group. The soldiers were able to maintain themselves in nitrogenous equilibrium on a dietary of poor protein

* Chittenden, " Physiological Economy in Nutrition," p. 43.
† Benedict and Carpenter : " Metabolism and Energy Transformations of Healthy Man during Rest."

value, the results showing that the daily excretion of the nitrogen of the urine ranged, over a period of five months for the different individuals, from 0·106 gramme up to 0·150 gramme per kilo of body weight. At the same time there was no great increase in the non-nitrogenous food—the fuel value never reaching 3,000 calories.

The third group consisted of eight students, all trained athletes. The men were under observation for a period of five months. No specific diet was imposed, as in the case of the soldiers of the Army Hospital Corps, but the men willingly cut down the intake of protein food, diminishing likewise in considerable measure the total volume of the food for the twenty-four hours. The results show that on an average this group excreted 8·81 grammes of nitrogen in the urine, as compared with an excretion of from 17 to 22 grammes when the men were living on their ordinary diet. Chittenden, again relying on the urinary nitrogen, gives the metabolized nitrogen of these eight students as varying from 0·108 to 0·165 gramme per kilo of body weight. The potential energy of the dietaries was not excessive—from 2,500 to 3,200 calories. It may be taken from the results of observations on these three groups that quantities of 56, 63, and 67 grammes protein in the diets were sufficient to maintain all these men in nitrogenous equilibrium. These quantities only represent 48 to 57 per cent. of Voit's standard.

The following table, compiled by v. Noorden, shows the different points brought to light in a manner easily grasped:

Groups.	No.	Average Weight.	Alteration in Weight.	Daily Nitrogen in Urine.	Nitrogen per Kilo.	Duration (Months).
		Kilos.	Kilos.	Grammes.	Grammes.	
I. Scientific workers	5	63·6	−2·9	7·52	0·12	6 to 9
II. Hospital corps	13	61·5	−1·7	7·90	0·13	6
III. Athletes ..	8	70·0	−3·5	8·81	0·13	5

Twenty out of the twenty-six subjects decreased in body weight in amounts varying from 1 to 9·2 kilos, the average loss of weight over the whole period being 2·5 kilos. The loss in weight was probably due largely to a decrease in body fat, but in some of the subjects there was certainly a fair degree of protein loss due to an insufficient amount of food.

Attempts were made to show that the subjects gained in body strength and in grace and ease in execution of movements. Some of the members of the Hospital Corps improved in health, and became free from certain disorders that had previously given trouble. From tests carried out this group showed an improvement of 100 per cent. in their dynamometric records. Even the athletes who had previously been in training showed an increase of 50 per cent. in muscular power.

As a general summary of his experimental results, Chittenden draws the conclusion that the need for protein food by adults may be fully met by a daily metabolism equal to an exchange of 0·12 gramme of nitrogen per kilo of body weight, provided the amount of non-nitrogenous food is sufficient to supply the energy requirements of the body. Hence for an average man weighing 70 kilos, or 154 pounds, 60 grammes of protein food daily would be amply sufficient to meet the needs of the body. "These, I believe, are perfectly trustworthy figures, with a reasonable margin of safety, and carrying perfect assurance of being really more than adequate to meet the true wants of the body, sufficient to supply all physiological demands for reserve protein, and able to cope with the erratic requirements of personal idiosyncrasies. It will be observed that such an intake of protein food daily is equal to one-half the Voit standard for a man of this weight."

In corroboration of Chittenden's findings there is the evidence afforded by a vegetarian married couple whose metabolism was investigated by Caspari and Glassner. The protein in the food varied from 33 to 49 grammes per day. Hamill and Schryver, from observations on the nitrogen excretion of scientific men in London, found that the protein of the diet was, on the average, about 70 grammes daily, a somewhat higher figure than Chittenden advocates, but considerably lower than the Voit standard.

Further, as has been shown on a large scale with regard to the teeming millions of Bengal, the great mass of the rice-eating inhabitants live on a protein intake that is even lower than that advocated by Chittenden, but which provides an identical nitrogenous metabolism per kilo of body weight—viz., about 0·12 gramme.

The most recent work* on the subject by Chittenden makes an attempt to prove that healthy men doing a moderate amount of work do not consume on an average the amount of protein food called for by the ordinary standards. With a view of obtaining evidence on this question, he made a large number of observations on healthy men, mostly young and vigorous students

* Chittenden, *British Medical Journal*, vol. ii., 1911.

of the University; some were athletic in build and tendencies, others slender, and inclined to take little physical exercise. The twenty-four hours' urine was collected, and the total amount of metabolized nitrogen determined, the subject taking his usual amount and character of food. One hundred and eight persons were so studied. The following are the points elucidated:

Number of Students.	Nitrogen of Urine.	Nitrogen Metabolized per Kilo of Body Weight.	Body Weight.
	Grammes.	Grammes.	Kilos.
108	12·87	0·194	66·2
Voit's standard	16·00	0·228	70·0

Chittenden draws the conclusion from these results that the 108 individuals selected at random from a large group of men were plainly taking a very much smaller amount of protein food than is generally considered essential for good health.

These men were apparently strong, healthy individuals, some of them indulging in vigorous athletic work, while as a group they represent the average type of vigorous manhood common to most University centres. He asks the question: "Are we to assume that this large group of men, taking on an average only 80 per cent. of the amount of protein food generally considered essential for health, were all in danger of nitrogen starvation? Certainly, if the Voit standard of 118 grammes of protein food represents the limit below which it is not safe for the average man to drop; then these individuals were living at a dangerously low level of nitrogen intake. Are we to assume that all these young men were unconsciously undermining their health, gradually destroying their vitality, and paving the way for the encroachment of disease through faulty habits of life."

We have quoted sufficiently from this interesting paper to show the line of argument adopted, but there are several points that appear to call for adverse criticism. These we shall deal with at once, reserving the consideration of Chittenden's results obtained from his three groups of subjects for the succeeding chapter.

1. Chittenden relies entirely on the nitrogen excreted in the urine as a measure of the nitrogenous metabolism; this is not an accurate method. Under conditions where the diet is uniform and does not vary from day to day, the average excretion of nitrogen in the urine over long periods may approximate closely

to the real nitrogenous metabolism; but for a short period of twenty-four hours, as in the observations on these 108 individuals, the urinary nitrogen could not be accepted as a true measure of the level of nitrogenous metabolism. It is well known to all who have worked on the elimination of nitrogen in the urine that, even with a uniform, non-varying dietary, there may be considerable variations in the daily excretion of urinary nitrogen; the diets of these students were freely selected, and doubtless varied from day to day.

The only true measure of the amount of nitrogen undergoing metabolism is the difference between the nitrogen intake and the loss of nitrogen to the body in the fæces. (The question of the nitrogen derived from the intestinal canal that has really been metabolized has already been discussed.)

The average quantity of 12.87 grammes given by Chittenden as the amount of metabolized nitrogen is therefore too low, as it makes no allowance for nitrogen that has undergone metabolism, but which has either been retained or has left the body in some way other than in the urine.

2. How are we to discover what the real average level of the nitrogenous metabolism of these 108 subjects is? In the latter part of the same paper Chittenden records the results of observations on six laboratory assistants over a period of 130 days. We have discussed this experiment already, and shown that under fairly similar conditions these six men, with an average intake of 12.02 grammes of nitrogen, metabolized 10.66 grammes, whilst only 9.16 grammes on the average appeared in the urine. That is, 1.5 grammes of nitrogen daily for each subject had actually undergone metabolism, but did not appear in either the urine or fæces. If we accept this average, which is based on Chittenden's figures, as the amount to be added to the nitrogen of the urine in order to arrive at the real nitrogenous metabolism, we get $12.87 + 1.50 = 14.37$ grammes of nitrogen per man daily. This works out at practically 90 grammes of metabolized protein as contrasted with 100 grammes provided in the ordinary standard, or 90 per cent. of its protein value.

3. Voit's dietary is fixed for an average man of 70 kilos doing an average amount of work, and provides 0.228 gramme of nitrogen per kilo of body weight. Now, Chittenden records details, in the paper referred to, of 33⅓ per cent. of the subjects under observation; the average body weight of these thirty-six persons was only 61.7 kilos, so that it would be expected they

THE PROTEIN REQUIREMENTS OF MANKIND 121

could live on considerably less protein than the individual of average physique, thus lowering the average amount of nitrogen metabolized for the whole series. However, leaving that aside, and taking notice only of the amount of nitrogen metabolized per kilo of body weight, we find for the 108 students the following facts as contrasted with Chittenden's results:

Number of Students.	Nitrogen Metabolized.	Nitrogen Metabolized per Kilo of Body Weight.	Body Weight.
	Grammes.	Grammes.	Kilos.
108 (Chittenden)	12·87	0·194	66·2
108 (corrected)	14·37	0·217	66·2
Voit's standard	16·00	0·228	70·0

That is, on an average, over the whole series there is a deficiency of 0·011 gramme of nitrogen per kilo of body weight compared with Voit's standard dietary. Considering that this result is obtained from a single day's collection of the urine, it must be acknowledged to approximate very closely to the ordinary accepted standards.

For these different reasons, it cannot be admitted that Chittenden has proved that these men, picked at random from a group of several thousands, habitually live on a much smaller amount of protein food than is called for by the commonly accepted standards. By working out the difference as contrasted with Voit's standard on a basis of nitrogen metabolized per kilo of body weight, 0·217 gramme is just over 95 per cent. of the metabolism permitted by Voit's dietary. This is a comparatively small difference, even were it based on results arrived at by strictly accurate methods, on which to attack the findings of physiologists all over the world, which findings show with almost universal unanimity that, where a free choice can be afforded, mankind consumes sufficient food materials to provide at least 100 grammes of protein on the average in his daily fare.

Incidentally, it shows that the subjects selected for observation, although they were considerably below the average weight of the normal American, only 66 kilos, the average American weighing 70 kilos, instinctively selected sufficient protein to maintain the level of their nitrogenous metabolism at very nearly the average height. They were not, therefore, "living at a dangerously low level of nitrogen intake, nor unconsciously undermining their health, and gradually destroying their vitality."

CHAPTER VI

THE MERITS AND DEMERITS OF DIETARIES POOR IN PROTEIN

It is very generally admitted at the present time that life can be maintained on a relatively low protein intake; all the accumulated evidence of experimental work on dietetics during recent years would corroborate the findings of the earlier workers on this point. Provided a certain minimum of protein be supplied, accompanied by sufficient potential energy, a fairly active life can be supported upon varying proportions of the three food elements.

This is no new discovery. As Spriggs points out, " Men have existed in the past, in the vicissitudes of wealth and poverty, freedom, and captivity, upon dietaries as varied in both quantity and quality as will ever be designed by experimentalists. The main object is, therefore, not to determine upon how much or how little a man can live, but what are the proportions of the foodstuffs upon which he is able to maintain the body in the highest degree of efficiency."

With regard to this latter point there is not the same agreement of opinion. Chittenden and his followers would have us believe that both the protein and potential energy of the usually accepted standards can be diminished very considerably with great benefit to the body, thus helping to increase man's greatest assets—viz., health, strength, capacity for work, and resistance to disease.

He further suggests that any excess of protein food over what may be regarded as the minimum amount on which nitrogenous equilibrium can be established, is so much waste, entailing unnecessary labour on the part of the organism, and at the same time exposing the tissues and organs to the possible deleterious action of this uncalled-for excess of nitrogenous waste products prior to their elimination from the body. The excretion of these bodies through the kidneys is supposed by Chittenden to be a special source of danger, and likely to result in permanent injury. Chittenden brings forward evidence from the observations on his three groups of subjects to corroborate these conclusions, and to show how greatly the different individuals benefited during the period when the protein intake was low.

As a general criticism, it may be said at once that there is no evidence whatsoever that the consumption of 100 grammes of protein is in any way injurious; there is no relationship between it and high arterial tension, arterial degeneration, and, least of all, between it and the incidence of granular kidney. We shall enter into this in more detail when dealing with the conditions that obtain in the Bengali; suffice it to say at present that there would appear to be a far greater danger—viz., that of malnutrition of the renal epithelium from the lowered or impoverished condition of the blood which accompanies, and is the direct result of, a low protein dietary.

This lower vitality permits of invasion of the kidneys by microorganisms which, under healthier conditions, would have been destroyed. Further, it may be well to point out that, according to Chittenden's views, all excess of nitrogen and amino-bodies beyond that necessary for endogenous metabolism—a few grammes daily—is rapidly converted into urea by the liver, and thus never has a chance of acting deleteriously on the organs and tissues; so that, on his own showing, the fear of injurious effects from the protein of diet is groundless. " *Per contra,*" as Hutchison puts it, "Chittenden has not succeeded in convincing me that a high protein standard is not possibly beneficial by its specific dynamic effect; that means that it is stimulant of metabolism that makes for vitality, and that for resistance to disease."

The general consensus of opinion amongst physiologists and clinicians is against Chittenden's conclusions: it cannot be said to be proved that any benefit to health results from a low protein dietary. In England the number of recruits refused admission into the army is very high, many of them being in poor condition from want of food. The poor, who suffer from defective supplies, are generally stunted, poorly developed, and, for years after reaching adult age, remain incapable of good bodily or mental work.* As we shall have occasion to point out, the quality and sufficiency of the food, and particularly a liberal allowance of

* Rowntree, quoted by Haig, *British Medical Journal,* vol. ii., 1911.

protein, has a marked influence on the physical development and welfare of a race. With regard to the protein element, v. Noorden asks the question : " That the organism may be injured by an overloading with the products of nitrogenous decomposition may be true in cases of disease, but is it true for the healthy individual ? Are the carnivora less healthy than the herbivora because they consume a larger quantity of flesh ? The danger resulting from the formation of toxins in the intestinal canal when large quantities of protein are taken seems scarcely to be founded on sufficiently strong evidence."

Chittenden's subjects all showed marked improvement in their general health and in bodily strength ; he claims these results as evidence of the merits of a low protein dietary. Against his conclusions it may be at once put forward that any healthy set of men placed under similar conditions on a diet rich in protein, instead of protein-poor, would, in all probability, have shown even better results. The great objection to the experiments is that they were carried out without controls.

The subjects were placed under almost ideal conditions for insuring the success of the investigations : they were made to lead regular lives ; their food was carefully chosen and properly cooked ; there was a total abstinence from alcohol, condiments, and indiscretions from consumption of rich foods, sweetmeats, etc. With a carefully regulated life such as these men were compelled to pursue, great improvement in health was only to be expected. Even in diseased conditions the regular routine of a sanatorium often transforms the bodily conditions in a comparatively short space of time. The 100 per cent. increase in strength shown by the members of the Army Hospital Corps is not of any importance further than to show that the men were in good health. Any man on a diet above the starvation limit who practised gymnastics for one and a half hours daily for six months would exhibit great improvement in strength, and in ease of execution of the required tests.

Benedict, in a critical examination of the data furnished by Chittenden regarding the absorption of protein exhibited by these eleven men of the Hospital Corps, brings to light one very important abnormality : During the three periods of the nitrogen balance—six, seven, and five days—all the men lived on practically the same ration. With normal healthy men eating the same kind and quantities of foodstuffs, practically identical quantities of protein will be absorbed by each individual—*i.e.*, the nitrogen lost to the body in the fæces will be nearly the same in all cases. The following are the results shown by these men:

No.	First Period: Intake, 49·4 grms. N.	Second Period: Intake, 66·7 grms. N.	Third Period: Intake, 43·1 grms. N.
1	7·68 grms. N. in fæces	12·39 grms. N. in fæces	9·37 grms. N. in fæces
2	10·24 ,, ,,	7·01 ,, ,,	9·38 ,, ,,
3	9·94 ,, ,,	16·15 ,, ,,	6·54 ,, ,,
4	9·61 ,, ,,	10·31 ,, ,,	10·11 ,, ,,
5	11·10 ,, ,,	13·71 ,, ,,	7·79 ,, ,,
6	12·10 ,, ,,	11·98 ,, ,,	8·30 ,, ,,
7	6·00 ,, ,,	8·47 ,, ,,	10·82 ,, ,,
8	10·75 ,, ,,	12·36 ,, ,,	9·40 ,, ,,
9	4·45 ,, ,,	13·46 ,, ,,	9·42 ,, ,,
10	8·26 ,, ,,	8·36 ,, ,,	11·46 ,, ,,
11	6·87 ,, ,,	7·18 ,, ,,	11·39 ,, ,,
12	4·56 ,, ,,	,, ,,	,, ,,

That is, during the first period, when 49·4 grammes of nitrogen were ingested by each individual, the nitrogen of the fæces was found to vary from 4·45 to 12·10 grammes. In the second period, with an intake of 66·7 grammes of nitrogen, the fæcal nitrogen varied from 7·01 to 16·15 grammes, and in the third period from 7·79 to 11·46 grammes, when the intake was 43·1 grammes of nitrogen.

These are certainly most surprising results, and entirely at variance with what would be expected to be the case with healthy men living on the same dietary. No such variations are usually met with under normal conditions, and, unless some fallacy has crept in during the isolation of the fæces for the stated periods, it is impossible to understand how such results were obtained. Benedict offers the explanation that the variations in digestibility of the same diet exhibited by the several individuals may possibly be due to the abnormally low protein intake having resulted in some disturbance of the alimentary tract, thus affecting its power of absorbing protein or the products of its tryptic digestion. Such a disturbance has been observed in animal experiments when the protein of the diet had been allowed to fall to a low level.

The figures shown above are of very great interest, and merit closer examination. From them the following variations in the absorption of protein by the different individuals on the same diet are obtained for the three periods:

THE PROTEIN ELEMENT IN NUTRITION

	First Period.	Second Period.	Third Period.
Nitrogen intake	49·4 grms.	66·7 grms.	43·1 grms.
Nitrogen absorption:			
Highest	91·0 per cent.	89·5 per cent.	82·0 per cent.
Lowest	75·5 ,,	75·8 ,,	73·4 ,,
Average	82·9 ,,	82·5 ,,	77·4 ,,

That is, extreme differences of 15·5, 13·7, and 8·6 per cent. in the absorption of protein are shown by the several subjects experimented with on the same diet during the three periods of nitrogen balance. That such large variations could be met with in normal healthy people is scarcely credible. Benedict quotes the results of forty-eight digestion experiments in which the same food was administered to thirty different individuals: Of 40 grammes of nitrogen ingested during a three-day experiment, 4·7 grammes were recovered in the fæces, whilst in the large majority of the experiments the variation was but 2 or 3 decigrammes on either side of the normal. It has now been well recognized that the percentage composition of the fæces under all diets is so uniform that some speak of foods as large or small fæces-producers, rather than as being capable of incomplete or complete absorption. In our work[*] on the dietaries of Bengal gaols, the percentages of nitrogen in the fæces was found to be fairly uniform under different conditions, whilst the total loss of nitrogen varied largely with the total weight of the stools passed. Also, over a very large number of observations made on prisoners[†] in the United Provinces, the percentage of nitrogen in the fæces was found to vary within very narrow limits, whatever the composition of the diet happened to be, whilst the total amount of fæcal matter and the total loss of nitrogen to the body varied directly with the weight of the dietary, so long as it was composed of the same food materials.

Some of the results obtained with batches of prisoners may be quoted to show how very little variation in the absorption of protein is met with in different individuals when on identical dietaries (see table, p. 127).

Although these diets are seemingly identical, the fact that the foodstuffs forming them differed considerably in chemical composition in the several gaols introduces extraneous factors in a

[*] Scientific Memoirs, Government of India, No. 37.
[†] Ibid., No. 48, pp. 177-185.

comparison of the figures for the different gaols. By taking the batches on the same diet in the individual gaols, we get strictly comparable results, and it will be evident how very similar the amounts of protein lost in the fæces are by different individuals when under the same dietetic conditions. Many similar results might be quoted to corroborate the finding of other experimenters, and to show that practically identical quantities of protein are absorbed by different individuals from the same diet, even when dealing with the highly vegetable dietaries of the tropics.

Gaol.	Diet.	Nitrogen of Fæces.
Agra Gaol	Wheat, dal, vegetables	5·96 grms. 5·60 ,,
Benares Gaol	,,	5·46 ,, 5·53 ,,
Naini Gaol	,,	5·05 ,, 5·00 ,,
Lucknow Gaol	,,	5·14 ,, 5·02 ,,

Another important point made evident from a scrutiny of Chittenden's figures is that the highest and lowest degree of protein absorption is not shown by the same individuals in the different periods. Thus, for example, take the case of No. 9: this man during the first period, with an intake of 49·06 grammes of nitrogen, loses only 4·45 grammes in the fæces; in the second period, with an intake of 66·48 grammes of nitrogen, he loses 13·46 grammes in the fæces; whilst in the third period, with an intake of 42·45 grammes of nitrogen (considerably less than during the first period), he loses 9·42 grammes in the fæces; *i.e.*, contrasted with the first period, this man, with 6·6 grammes of nitrogen less in his diet, actually loses over twice as much of its nitrogen in the fæces. This means a protein absorption during the first period of 91 per cent., and during the third barely 78 per cent. Similarly, reference to the figures for Nos. 1, 4, 7, 9, 10, and 11 will show that there was a greater loss of nitrogen in the fæces during the third period, with an intake of 43 grammes, than during the first period with 49 grammes.

Comparison of the results given for the first and second periods, and for the second and third periods, show very great irregularities also. Thus, as a last example, we may take the figures for No. 2: with an intake of 49 grammes of nitrogen, he loses

10·24 grammes in the fæces; with an intake of 66 grammes, he loses 7 grammes in the fæces; and with an intake of 43 grammes of nitrogen, he loses 9·38 grammes in the fæces. Results such as these defy explanation, except on the assumption that they are not the records of a normally working organism, or that, owing to the difficulty in obtaining accurate collection of the fæces, except when the subjects are under constant supervision, the fæcal nitrogen figures do not represent the total loss of nitrogen in some, at least, of the recorded observations.

Taking into consideration the amount of vegetable material in the composition of the dietaries during the three periods, it would appear very probable that the higher figures given for the loss of nitrogen in the fæces are more likely to be correct than the smaller quantities. It is for this reason that it appears to us probable that the total quantity of fæces passed during the periods by some of the subjects was not collected in full amount. It may be, on the other hand, as Benedict indicates, that the higher figures given for the fæcal nitrogen are abnormal, owing to diarrhœa, or a low degree of protein absorption set up by some disturbance in the digestive powers of the alimentary tract, and which is the result of existence on a low level of protein metabolism. Whatever the true interpretation of Chittenden's figures may be, the fact remains that they are most irregular, and in the present state of our knowledge cannot be accepted as evidence of the merits of a low protein form of dietary. The fact that only a very small proportion of the men showed a positive nitrogen balance during the first and third periods would make it evident that the metabolism of 50 grammes of protein per day was not sufficient for the needs of the body, even with an average fuel value of 2,830 calories.

An examination of the results of the nitrogen eliminated in the urine gives equally discordant results. The figures are given in the table on p. 129.

Here, again, wide variations are recorded in the urinary nitrogen of the different individuals on the same diet: in the first period the limits are 40·12 grammes and 58·07 grammes; in the second period they are 42·37 and 56·60 grammes; whilst in the third period quantities of 28·89 grammes and 38·32 grammes are found. On the whole, however, the figures are more uniform than those given for the fæces, and it would therefore appear probable that the subject of the experiment took more care in the saving and collection of the urine than in the case of the fæces.

Subjects.	First Period.	Second Period.	Third Period.
Intake of nitrogen	49·40 grms.	66·70 grms.	43·10 grms.
1	45·13 ,,	50·74 ,,	35·21 ,,
2	44·54 ,,	55·32 ,,	33·19 ,,
3	42·66 ,,	42·37 ,,	*28·89 ,,
4	44·70 ,,	55·46 ,,	32·55 ,,
5	48·07 ,,	50·11 ,,	31·27 ,,
6	48·31 ,,	49·04 ,,	38·32 ,,
7	47·33 ,,	†55·10 ,,	36·81 ,,
8	40·12 ,,	49·90 ,,	32·52 ,,
9	58·64 ,,	56·60 ,,	37·15 ,,
10	45·07 ,,	49·08 ,,	35·41 ,,
11	46·98 ,,	†44·53 ,,	32·49 ,,

That such wide variations should occur in the elimination of nitrogen in the urine with different individuals living on the same diet shows how little reliance can be placed on the urinary nitrogen as a measure of the total nitrogenous metabolism. With single subjects over short periods it is a most unreliable method, even when a correction is added for the nitrogen metabolized, but which does not appear in the urine. With batches of men over relatively long periods, the average quantity of nitrogen excreted in the urine may be relied on to some extent, when all sources of fallacy are guarded against and provided for.

A summary of the results obtained by Chittenden with his eleven subjects shows—

Subjects.	First Period.	Second Period.	Third Period.
Average N. intake per man	8·23 grms.	9·53 grms.	8·62 grms.
,, (urine) ,,	7·75 ,,	7·25 ,,	6·79 ,,
,, (fæces) ,,	1·41 ,,	1·66 ,,	1·95 ,,

That is, there is actually a lower amount of nitrogen excreted in the urine during the second period, when the nitrogen intake was 9·53 grammes, than during the first period, when it was only 8·23 grammes; further, the quantity of nitrogen lost in the fæces was higher in the third period than in the second period, although the nitrogen intake was considerably less.

We may conclude this examination of Chittenden's results by

* Corrected for five days.   † Corrected for seven days.

pointing out that on an average during the second period, when the men showed a positive nitrogen balance, the urinary nitrogen points to a protein absorption of 76 per cent., whilst the true amount is really 82·5 per cent. The absorption of protein for the subjects individually, on the other hand, based, according to Chittenden's method, on the urinary nitrogen, shows much greater variations : thus, No. 3 would seemingly show an absorption of less than 64 per cent., the real amount being 75·3 per cent., according to the figures given for the total intake and the loss of nitrogen in the fæces.

On the whole, while the figures recorded by Chittenden for the balance period and those given for the elimination of nitrogen in the urine during the several months of observation are open to a considerable amount of criticism, the fact remains that these men existed for months, if not on the low amount of nitrogen per kilo of body weight that Chittenden found, at least on dietaries that would appear to have contained very much less protein than that provided in Voit's standard.* It must be accepted also that during the period of five months the men showed no signs of diminished strength or loss of bodily vigour.

The studies carried out with eight athletes demonstrate that this class can very materially reduce the quantity of protein in their diet, and, at the same time, gain enormously in strength, and win in intercollegiate and other athletic contests. As these men were in training before the change of diet took place, the evidence afforded by their improvement in strength and physical condition is of greater importance on the merits of a low protein dietary than the increase in physical powers recorded in the case of the soldiers.

It would appear from the opinions expressed by those in charge of the training of these men that the good results obtained are entirely to be ascribed to the lowered protein intake, whilst any ill-effects can always be explained away as due to some cause other than diet. Thus the winning of two championships is specially suggested as being due to the restricted diet. Another man won points for the first time ; others showed no falling off, or were actually believed to have improved their position as athletes. It is reported that all lost in weight, some very considerably; but that is made light of, and even regarded as a condition devotedly to be wished. Considering that all these men

* For more recent information on this point, see note on p. 148.

were in hard training before the change of diet occurred, it is open to doubt whether the loss of weight is to be regarded as of little consequence in estimating the ultimate effects of a low protein dietary. This is the very condition most evident in the races of India, whose dietary for generations and centuries has been deficient in absorbable protein; the body weight is very low, in spite of the diet containing considerable amounts of carbonaceous matter and being of great caloric value. The great deficiency is met with in the muscular and protoplasmic tissues; nothing could be more remarkable than the miserable condition of the musculature of those races whose dietary permits of a protein metabolism complying with the standard laid down by Chittenden as sufficient to meet the nitrogenous requirements of the body. We believe—and the facts as met with on a large scale in India warrant our belief—that, while it may be possible for the average man or athlete to carry on for a time without any very striking ill-effects on a low protein dietary, sooner or later a breakdown will come, for which, doubtless, there may be the most plausible non-dietetic explanations to offer, but which, in truth, is the outcome of existence on a protein intake insufficient to maintain the body in a high state of efficiency.

The conclusions Chittenden draws from the work done on these eight athletes—and, indeed, the same applies to his soldier group also—would be more convincing if the results had been controlled, or even if there had been comparative tests with a similar set of athletes on a liberal protein dietary. There must be records of similar tests made in the progress of athletic training during previous years, and it seems a pity, if such exist, that they have not been made use of as a standard of comparison.

There is no doubt, however, that the reports on these men, while on the restricted diet, show marked increase in strength and skill in carrying out the tests. Considering the great interest taken in intercollegiate contests, it is all the more remarkable, if such marked benefit followed so rapidly on this dietetic alteration, that similar changes have not been insisted on by trainers and willingly accepted by athletes, not only at Yale, but all over the world. Nothing of the kind has occurred. It is generally believed that even the men, who are reported to have benefited so greatly from the new ideas on the protein requirements, returned at once to their former diet as soon as the experiment was discontinued.

We may conclude the examination of Chittenden's three classes of experiment by summing up the objections put forward to them, and to any general adoption of dietaries containing the low level of protein he advocates :

1. The method of basing the protein requirements of the body on the average amount of nitrogen eliminated in the urine gives too low a result for the protein metabolism per kilo of body weight.

2. The very great variations recorded for the digestibility and absorption of protein from identical diets for the individual members of his second group—men of the hospital corps—can either be explained on the basis of malnutrition of the intestinal epithelium, the result of a diet poor in protein, or by failure of the men to collect all the fæces passed each day, so that the total amount included in the analyses was too low. For several reasons we believe the latter to be the more likely explanation. If this should be the explanation, it must throw a certain amount of doubt on the collection of the daily urine for the five months during which this experiment was carried out. Any loss of urine would mean a seemingly lower level of nitrogenous metabolism than was actually the case. It is well known how difficult it is to save all the excretions, except where the most rigid precautions are taken. In the work in India we found it absolutely necessary to confine prisoners under observation to solitary cells, in order to insure the complete collection of the urine and fæces. This criticism would not apply to Chittenden's first and third groups of subjects, who were educated men, and who would fully understand the importance of saving the excreta in full.

3. Whilst one feels bound to accept the figures stated for the daily intake of nitrogen in the dietaries published throughout Chittenden's book, at the same time one cannot help feeling that they would have been much more satisfactory if the nitrogen of those dietaries had been computed from analyses of the dry food materials used, before being cooked, instead of being estimated by means of factors for the percentage of nitrogen in cooked food. The percentage of moisture in any cooked food may vary very considerably from day to day; this would be specially marked with the more or less vegetarian types of diet Chittenden was compelled to have recourse to in order to keep down the protein content.

Apart from these technical objections which could be easily overcome, there has been considerable mass of criticism levelled at Chittenden's results, and the more remote effects of dietaries low in protein. Hutchison* summarizes some of these, and Crichton-Browne† discusses many others in detail:

1. While a low standard of protein intake may be adopted with apparent impunity for considerable periods, it does not follow that it can safely be pursued indefinitely. Excess of protein is regarded as a margin of safety in increasing the general tone of the system and the resistance to disease. Just as chronic excesses in diet are slow in exacting their penalties, so a subliminal diet may also be tardy in manifesting its untoward effects.

It is generally recognized that abrupt changes in the daily food are very liable to produce gastro-intestinal trouble and failure in health. It is quite possible that radical changes, even when gradually introduced, may have ill-effects of an insidious nature long before there is any obvious breakdown in health.

2. Existence at the lower limits of protein metabolism undoubtedly results in a wasting of the nitrogenous tissues and fluids of the body during every special call or demand for increased effort. This disintegrated tissue may take weeks to replace, and thus convalescence from illness may be prolonged and recovery rendered incomplete.

3. The effects of a diminished protein intake on the race is of far greater importance than on the individual. The experiences gained in India are specially interesting from this point of view, and will be fully discussed presently. Suffice it at present to say, that those people whose dietary affords a low level of protein metabolism are, so far as our knowledge goes, of poor physique, wanting in stamina, and lacking in the manly quantities that are essential in commanding and maintaining the respect of the more virile races.

4. Chittenden's claim, that the elimination of crystalline nitrogenous bodies through the kidneys places upon these organs an unnecessary burden, which is liable to endanger their integrity, and possibly result in serious injury, in so far as it applies to the ordinary accepted standard, cannot be substantiated, and is opposed to universal experience.

Many other points might be raised, some of which we shall discuss in detail later. One very important subject is the bearing of a low protein dietary on the susceptibility to disease. We have

* Hutchison, " Food and the Principles of Dietetics," p. 24.
† Sir J. Crichton-Browne, " Parsimony in Nutrition," 1909

already referred to the marvellous results that followed an increase in protein of the ration of the Japanese Navy. The importance of a liberal dietary in the treatment of certain pathological conditions is well recognized by the medical profession. The lymphocytosis that accompanies digestion has been shown to be much increased by a diet of raw meat, and the modern methods of combating tuberculosis make use of a regimen in which protein is in liberal quantities as the best means of arresting the disease. The marked success that has attended the Weir-Mitchell treatment, one element of which is high protein feeding, is acknowledged on all sides. According to Chittenden's ideas, this heavy protein intake, combined with rest, should set up all manner of ailments. The results are exactly the opposite: the nutrition of the patient is restored and health returns. In India, the home of epidemic diseases, famines or years of scarcity never fail to be accompanied by outbreaks of infections which pick out with unfailing regularity those who have become enfeebled from want of proper food. Examples of the great importance of a high level of nutrition in decreasing the susceptibility to infection could easily be largely multiplied, but enough has been said at present to give us pause before accepting the conclusions arrived at by Chittenden from experiments largely laboratory in nature, and carried out under relatively artificial conditions.

It has been estimated that over 30 per cent. of the population of the large towns in England and other countries are in a condition of under-nourishment from chronic under-feeding; the consequences of this is not "increased vigour, improved health, and exhilaration of spirits, but weakness, misery, and degeneration." The lethargic appearance of the protein-starved, rice-eating populace of parts of the tropics is in marked contrast to the alert and energetic demeanour of those who, living under absolutely identical conditions as regards climate and customs, are able to afford a dietary in which a sufficient amount of absorbable protein is present.

In connection with this thought, the following excerpt from a work by Nietzsche may be quoted: "When a profound dislike for existence gets the upper hand, the after-effects of a great error in diet of which a people has been long guilty comes to light. The spread of Buddhism (not its origin) is thus to a considerable extent dependent on the excessive and almost exclusive rice fare of the Indians, and on the universal enervation that results therefrom. . . . The increased prevalence of rice-eating impels to the use of opium and narcotics. . . . It also impels, however, in its more subtle after-effects, to modes of thought and feeling which operate narcotically."

Dr. I. M. Mullick,* in a study of the medical aspect of student life in Calcutta, states that 50 per cent. are melancholic, pessimistic, never enjoy life properly, this condition arising both from actual want as well as from imaginary evils. In dilating on their ill-developed, weak, and defective physique, he ascribes the important cause to diet and an insufficient amount of easily assimilable protein. As a result of protein starvation, the muscles are enfeebled and the body does not attain its full development and growth ; these effects on the race are most lasting and dangerous. Hence the preponderance of so many infectious diseases in the land, which are largely predisposed to by the low resisting power of the system.

We may now refer to some other observations and investigations bearing on the merits or demerits of the low protein standard advocated by Chittenden. The very interesting and instructive knowledge, gained from experiences in the local and convict prisons of England, with the dietaries in force before the introduction of the present scales, is of special importance :

No. 1 diet provided—
Protein .. .. 57 grms.
Carbohydrates .. 341 ,, } Caloric value, 1,464 calories.
Fat .. .. 19 ,,

—*i.e.*, practically identical with Chittenden's protein standard.

No. 2 diet provided—
Protein .. .. 70 grms.
Carbohydrates .. 385 ,, } Caloric value, 1,684 calories.
Fat .. .. 21 ,,

—*i.e.*, considerably above Chittenden's standard in protein.

Convict diet for light labour provided—
Protein .. .. 133 grms.
Carbohydrates .. 478 ,, } Caloric value, 2,398 calories.
Fat .. .. 44 ,,

—*i.e.*, greatly in excess of the amount of protein Chittenden would consider amply sufficient.

These dietaries had been in force for twenty years, and were regarded as physiologically correct and amply sufficient. However, when the subject came before Parliament, a terrible indict-

* Dr. Mullick, *Calcutta Medical Journal*, April, 1909.

ment was brought against them by members who had had practical experience of their ill-effects. A committee was appointed to examine and report on their adequacy, with the result that they were condemned, and new scales—considerably more liberal—were introduced.

It was clearly proved that Diets 1 and 2 were absolutely insufficient to satisfy the pangs of hunger, and were injurious to health, as indicated by a loss of weight. Many suffered from gastro-intestinal disturbances, thus conforming with the experiences of Munk and Rosenheim when feeding dogs on a low protein dietary. In this connection it may be pointed out that intestinal disorders are exceedingly prevalent in India; but they are very much more common amongst the rice-eating, protein-starved populace than amongst those whose dietary contains some of the superior cereals.

Evidence was produced to show that prisoners would go to almost any extreme to satisfy the pangs of hunger. Men would gather and eat snails, eat the putrid marrow of bones, pick up fragments of candles, purposely made offensive so as not to be eaten, wipe them with their clothes, and eat them. These were the immediate effects of diets Chittenden believes amply sufficient; the remote consequences were probably still more glaring and far-reaching. The number who left the prisons permanently broken in health as the results of dietetic privation and impaired nutrition will never come to light, but we are justified in assuming, in the light of the recognized influence of privation in predisposing to tuberculosis, that many on this account fell victims to the tubercle bacillus.

One of the most valuable studies of prison dietaries is that made by Dr. J. C. Dunlop for the Prison Commission of Scotland. His standards are based on careful investigations carried out on scientific lines, and upon actual experience have been found satisfactory. Starting with the amount of food necessary to nourish the body, the quantity is modified according to the different conditions of the individuals to be fed. The more important dietaries are given in the table on p. 137.

Dr. Dunlop found that prisoners, when reduced below 3,500 calories of food energy per day, 82 per cent. of those of average size lost weight.

In France the prison dietary provides—

Protein .. .. 94 grms. ⎫
Carbohydrates .. .. .. 374 ,, ⎬ 2,074 calories,
Fat .. .. 22 ,, ⎭

or over one-third more protein than the Chittenden standard; yet Dr. Gautier, the greatest French authority on dietetics, states that it is too poor in protein, even for a man who does not work. He lays it down that a man on hard labour should be provided with 135 grammes of protein and from 500 to 700 grammes of carbonaceous material—more than double the Chittenden standard.

DUNLOP'S STANDARDS.

Different Classes of Prisoners.	Protein.	Fat.	Carbohydrates.	Energy Value.
	Grms.	Grms.	Grms.	Calories.
Ordinary male prisoners	120	38	550	3,100
,, female ,,	96	30	440	2,480
,, ,, ,, (nursing)	105	54	482	2,910
Male prisoners unemployed	90	30	440	2,400
Female ,, ,,	72	23	330	1,860
Male convicts, hard labour	150	65	550	3,500
,, ,, light ,,	120	50	550	3,200
Female convicts	100	41	440	2,600
Punishment diet	90	30	440	2,400
,, ,, (subsistence)	64	21	341	1,850

It may be concluded, therefore, from the knowledge gained from a study of prison dietaries, that the results do not bear out Chittenden's contentions.

Other points bearing on this subject have been admirably summarized by Spriggs in his article on the results of experimental work on diet.* He quotes Darwin's remarks on his visit to the Chilian copper mines. The ore had to be carried up a 450-feet shaft in loads of 200 pounds. The men were pale, and some of them with but little muscular development. They were fed on beans and bread; the men preferred bread, which was a luxury; but the masters, finding they could not work so hard upon this, were accustomed to treat them like horses, and make them eat the beans. In beans 20 per cent. of the energy is in the form of protein, whereas in bread only about 12 per cent. is present as such.

Livingstone records that the grain-eating tribes of Central Africa could not endure fatigue so well as the beef-eaters, who scorned the idea of ever being tired.

Dr. Zieman, from a careful study of the hygienic conditions of tropical Africa, states that one of the most influential of the

* Spriggs, " A System of Diet and Dietetics." Sutherland, 1908.

causes which tend to diminish the number and impoverish the physique of the coloured races is not over- but under-feeding.

On the other hand, Irving Fisher claims that a decrease in the protein element of the diet is favourable to endurance. He carried out a series of feeding experiments on nine healthy students, lasting for five months, with endurance tests at the beginning, middle, and end of the period. During this period the total calories of the daily ration had fallen 25 per cent., the protein 40 per cent., and the fresh food 80 per cent. Six simple gymnastic tests were employed, such as raising the body on the toes, holding the arms horizontally, raising and lowering the dumb-bell.

The endurance was found to be much greater at the end than at the beginning of the experiment. It appears to us these tests are not of the slightest value, unless the nine students were under constant supervision, and it could be definitely stated that they did not practise the required tests in the intervals. These observations, again, were carried out without controls, and it is more than probable that the results recorded are easily explained as due to practice by the students in order to make the experiment a success.

On the other hand, the students showed loss of strength in the grip and loss of weight. These ill-effects are attributed to over-study or other causes, but the increase in endurance was, of course, entirely due to the low protein dietary. Spriggs remarks that these considerations do not inspire confidence in the diet.

Fortunately, in the interests of truth, we are able to place on record some evidence of very recent date, which appears to us to be of considerable value in appraising the effects of a low protein dietary. It has already been shown that the average Indian student in Calcutta lives on a protein metabolism closely approximating the Chittenden standard, whilst Anglo-Indian and Eurasian students receive dietaries more nearly approaching Voit's standard. We shall have more to say on the effects of this difference later, but at present a brief account of the comparative tests afforded by the intercollegiate athletic sports in Calcutta will be given.

Twelve colleges entered representative teams to compete in the different events. The very great majority of the students attending these colleges are Indian, the Anglo-Indian and Eurasian probably not exceeding 2 per cent. of the total number.

Despite the small community to select from, the Anglo-Indian and Eurasian were largely chosen by the athletic clubs to represent their colleges. The results of the tests, which included the usual events—100 yards, hurdles, 220 yards, 440 yards, half, and mile races, broad and high jump, tug-of-war, etc.—are very striking. The Anglo-Indians and Eurasians were first and second in nine out of twelve events: the prizes for the competitors who won most events, awarded on points, were both secured by Anglo-Indian and Eurasian; the challenge shield offered for the college whose representatives scored the greatest number of points was won by the college which was almost entirely represented by Anglo-Indians and Eurasians—in fact, the Indian students were outclassed in almost every test, whether of strength or skill.

These results are even more remarkable than they appear at first sight. The students of Anglo-Indian and Eurasian extraction enter college much younger than the Indian students, and are not fully developed until their last two years in residence. The Indian students have large numbers to choose from, and great interest is taken in sports of all kinds, each of the colleges having flourishing athletic, cricket, football, and other clubs. Yet, despite their comparatively insignificant numbers, and their relatively immature age, these Anglo-Indian and Eurasian students were markedly superior to their Indian fellow-students in tests that were strictly comparable. It is not to be understood, however, that all Anglo-Indians and Eurasians develop into men superior in physique to the Indians; the properly fed do, but the cities, and particularly the hospitals, are full of miserable specimens who, owing to their poverty-stricken condition, are unable to afford other than the cheapest food materials, and who live on dietaries no better than, if as good as, the poorer classes of Indians.

Other points of evidence bearing on the question have been put forward. Thus Benedict states, from the results of numerous dietary studies made with different classes of people living under different conditions, that it has been observed that with communities a generally low condition of mental and physical efficiency, thrift, and commercial success is coincident with a low proportion of protein in the diet. He cites the negro and poor white of the South, and the Italian labourer of Southern Italy, all of whom partake of diets relatively low in protein, and states that their sociological condition and commercial enterprise are on a par with their diet. Yet, when these people are fed on a higher protein plane, their productive power increases markedly.

All the successful races have habitually consumed protein far in excess of the amount Chittenden believes sufficient, whereas those who have adhered to a low protein standard have not progressed physically, mentally, or morally. The poorer races of India and the tropics illustrate this truth, and show that the conquering races and nations are all high protein feeders. Chittenden would have us believe that they are high protein feeders because they are conquerors, but the facts do not bear out his contention.

We shall now consider briefly the knowledge gained on this subject from experimental work done on animals, reserving for the following chapters the more recent observations and investigations made on some of the different tribes and races of India.

Experiments on Animals.

Numerous studies have been made on the effects of decreasing the protein element in the food of different animals.

Munk, Rosenheim, Hagemann, and Jägerroos, have made investigations bearing on the question of the reduction of the protein in the diet of dogs. Rosenheim and Munk obtained bad results when the protein element was decreased to 2 grammes of protein per kilo of body weight; the animals suffered from digestive troubles, such as vomiting and loss of appetite. They showed very defective absorption of food, and after a few months died in an apathetic condition.

Jägerroos, taking special precautions, was able to keep two bitches alive for six and a half months on an intake of less than 2 grammes of protein per kilo of body weight. Both these dogs died rapidly, not, as Jägerroos states, from the results of protein starvation and inanition, but from an acute infection contracted after the premature delivery of one of them: in all probability due to a lowered resistance to infection from the ill-effects of poor feeding.

Chittenden, in a report on experiments completed on six dogs, traverses the results reported by previous investigators, and states that they were not due to the effects of low protein, or to a diminished consumption of non-nitrogenous food, but are to be ascribed mainly to non-hygienic conditions, or to a lack of care and physiological good sense in the prescription of a narrow dietary not suited to the habits and needs of this class of animal.

Chittenden's experiments on dogs were carried out under the most favourable circumstances to insure the successful issue of the investigation. The animals were nursed and tended in the most painstaking manner, and every source of danger was guarded against. It must be acknowledged that he has accomplished what no previous experimenter had been able to do—viz., maintain dogs in fair health and keep them alive for varying periods of time over six months on dietaries providing less than 2 grammes of protein and 80 calories of fuel value per kilo of body weight.

As an example of the thorough and whole-hearted methods Chittenden has made use of throughout all his researches on nutrition, nothing he has done shows more clearly his infinite capacity for taking pains than the prolonged experiments devised and carried out with such scrupulous care on these dogs. However, even his methods and results in this experiment have been unfavourably criticized. It has been pointed out * :

1. He proves too much, for in several instances, as the nitrogen and fuel value of the diet per kilo of body weight became reduced during the course of the experiment, his dogs actually increased in weight. No. 5 dog increased from 15·5 to 20 kilos on reduction of the nitrogen from 0·54 to 0·26 gramme, and the fuel value from 87 to 65 calories per kilo of body weight. It almost appears as if nitrogen in the diet were entirely superfluous.

2. No notice is taken of the build and shape of the animal, although the body surface, and consequently the amount of heat lost by radiation, must have varied enormously.

3. The kind of dog is not specified, which is a point of great importance, as different kinds of dogs are habituated to different kinds of diet. Some dogs get practically no meat ; others, like the coursing greyhound, are trained on the best beef and mutton.

4. They led a placid and cloistered existence. For ten days in each month they lived in the metabolism cage, and for the remainder of the time practically in kennels.

5. Not until a pack of foxhounds have got satisfactorily through a winter's work on Chittenden's reduced diet can his

* Sir J. Crichton-Browne, " Parsimony in Nutrition."

experiments be accepted as anything more than a curious physiological feat.

6. The experiences of zoological gardens, farmers, breeders of cattle, horses, and domestic pets, are all quoted against Chittenden's conclusions. In fact, he would appear to stand alone against the world in his stringent ideas on protein economy.

On reading carefully through the accounts of these experiments, two other points appear to be worthy of attention. One is the exceedingly small amount of nitrogen lost to the body in the fæces, being often less than that given for the nitrogen "lost through hair." Thus, for the total of the eleven periods recording the nitrogen balances of subject No. 5, the nitrogen lost in the fæces amounts to 5·93 grammes, whilst that lost "through hair" is 5·44 grammes. Another point is that the protein absorption from the dietaries made use of does seem to have fallen as the experiment proceeded.

Taking subject No. 5 again—the only one concerning which we have any details—we find the following results:

Diet I.

Meat	172 grms.
Cracker dust	124 "
Lard	72 "

Absorption of protein, 91 per cent.

Diet II.

Meat	70 grms.
Cracker dust	124 "
Lard	72 "

Absorption of protein, 93 per cent.

—*i.e.*, although the highly absorbable protein of meat was reduced from 172 to 70 grammes, the protein absorption from the diet increased by 2 per cent.

Diet IV.

Meat	69 grms.
Bread	166 "
Lard	80 "

Absorption of protein, 91 per cent.

Diet VI.

Meat	70 grms.
Cracker dust	158 "
Lard	60 "

Absorption of protein, 86 per cent.

Contrasting the result shown by Diet VI. with the protein absorption from Diet II., a fall of 7 per cent. would not be expected, unless the intestinal power of absorption had become less efficient as the dieting proceeded. Chittenden, while admitting that the utilization of nitrogen becomes less complete in the later dietaries, attempts to explain it away as being due to a decrease in the quantity of readily digestible meat and an increase in the vegetable material of these diets. As will be evident from the diets selected above, this explanation will not cover the facts. Diets II., IV., and VI. are practically identical in their absorbability, yet the dog shows considerable variations in the quantity of protein he was able to utilize. It is therefore not quite clear from these experiments that the absorptive function of the intestinal epithelium did not suffer to some extent by the protein content of the dietaries remaining at so low a level for many months. This would be in harmony with the conclusions arrived at by Munk and Rosenheim from a similar series of experiments, and would militate against the view that a material reduction of the protein in dietaries is to the welfare of the body.

All these experiments on dogs are open to the criticism that the dog is a carnivorous animal, and that the results are therefore not directly transferable to man. We shall now refer to some experiments on animals that are more nearly allied in food habits to man. The most important of these are the investigations made into the effects of feeding swine on a low and on a high protein dietary respectively.

The digestive organs of the pig are regarded as being closely comparable to those of man, and the pig, being an omnivorous animal, like man, is not open to the same objection as the dog in estimating the merits or demerits of a low protein dietary. Benedict, quoting from Shutt's valuable and interesting paper,* states that extensive investigations on "soft" pork show conclusively that when hogs are fed on a low protein diet—i.e., Indian corn—the pork is of very inferior quality; while if the protein content of the diet is raised by the addition of skim milk, legumes, or other nitrogenous materials, the quality of the pork is very markedly improved.

Canadian pork butchers find also that the intestines of hogs fed on low protein rations tear more easily when the carcass is dressed—that is, the intestines are not so firm. This would appear analogous to the condition described by Munk and Rosenheim as occurring in the intestines of the dogs they investigated in their feeding experiments with dietaries deficient in protein. A bad quality of pork is also produced when the diet is excessively high in protein, so that swine are unusually sensitive to marked alterations in the protein content of the diet.

* Shutt, Bulletin No. 38, Department of Agriculture, Ottawa, Canada.

These Canadian observations have been corroborated by the work of Skinner* in Indiana, who fed hogs on a low protein dietary of Indian meal. This diet caused impairment of the digestive capacity, which became more apparent the longer the diet was continued. It resulted in "poor appetites, light bone, deficient development in valuable portions of the carcass, and a general state of unthrift, as shown by the hair, skin, and hungry look of the animals." The addition of one-sixth of the amount of the ration in materials rich in protein resulted in normal growth and a healthy condition.

A similar series of experiments have been carried out by Professor Haecker on herbivorous animals. Benedict, quoting from unpublished results, remarks that herbivora being accustomed to diets relatively low in protein, a further decrease would be expected to be accompanied by less marked disturbances, which might take a considerable time to develop, than in the case of carnivora or omnivora.

Haecker's investigations were carried out with the view of determining, from an economical standpoint, to what extent the amount of protein could be decreased with safety and economy.

Two groups of cows of ten in each group were fed for a period of three years, one group on a diet containing the normal proportion of protein, the other on a much lower protein ration. No ill-effects appear to have been noticeable for some time, although the second group had lost somewhat in weight. During the first part of the third winter both groups did well, but by January the cows receiving the low protein dietary began to fail. By March 13 it became absolutely necessary to increase the proportion of protein, as the cows had become very thin in flesh, and their coats dry and harsh—a well-recognized indication of under-nutrition.

It is particularly worthy of attention that the effects of a low protein dietary on the pigs and cows was very gradual, but, nevertheless, led in time to a general deterioration of health. The importance of this in appraising the merits of dietaries low in protein for man cannot be over-estimated. It demonstrates clearly that experiments with diets of low protein content, to be conclusive, should last for years, as the beneficial effects of previous high protein feeding may be persistent and prolonged.

* Skinner, Indiana Agriculture Experimental Station, Bulletin No. 108.

It may be concluded from the evidence so far adduced that a considerable mass of experimental facts and deductions from accurate observation have been accumulated, which, in their general bearing, militate very strongly against the conclusion that a marked reduction in the protein element of the average diet is either necessary or desirable. We have summarized some of the technical and more general objections that a critical examination of Chittenden's investigations on his three groups of subjects would make apparent. The object of our scrutiny of Chittenden's work and of the different points brought forward has been to determine whether the records demonstrate any evidence of ill-effects due to dietetic changes. Several such demerits have been pointed out, and others suggested.

When a survey is made of Chittenden's brilliant piece of work, it must be admitted that he has made out a very strong case. He has been the first to show that man can live and do a certain amount of work on an intake of protein much below the ordinary accepted standards without increasing—indeed, with a considerable diminution of—the fuel value of the diet. While accepting this finding, we have shown that there remains a considerable degree of doubt whether his subjects did live during the months of experimentation on the low protein dietaries the urinary nitrogen would indicate.

As pointed out, serious sources of error may have resulted, in the absence of supervision, from the failure of the different individuals to collect and surrender the full amount of the daily urine and to adhere strictly to the diet prescribed. Even during the periods of balance, when the food partaken of was accurately weighed and its nitrogen content estimated, the fact that this nitrogen was computed from certain factors for the percentage of protein of cooked foods leaves open a considerable loophole of error. The great irregularity displayed by the individuals of his second group in their utilization of the protein while on absolutely identical diets does not tend to inspire confidence in the accuracy with which the members of the Hospital Corps collected the fæces; or, if this view be doing them an injustice, and the figures given are correct, then the varying absorption of protein they indicate can only be explained as an ill-effect of the abnormally low protein dietary—seriously injuring the absorptive function of the intestinal epithelium.

These doubts are strengthened when the figures for the fuel

value of the diets are taken into consideration. Chittenden would not only lower the protein standard, but would likewise decrease materially the potential energy of diets. Whatever may be the true physiological requirements of the body for protein in maintaining it in a thorough condition of efficiency, there can be no doubt concerning the recognized fact that the total energy requirements must be met by the oxidation of the food partaken of, unless the organized tissues or reserve materials are to be drawn on. Benedict, from a series of brilliant experiments, carried out by means of the respiration calorimeter, has shown that a man of average size, weighing 66 kilos, and at rest within the calorimeter, in twenty-four hours expends about 2,270 calories. The average individual under ordinary conditions, but not at work, would require more; whilst the same individual engaged in labour will dissipate large amounts of energy in proportion to the work done. Quantities up to 600 calories per hour have been recorded as the output of energy by a professional bicycle rider.

It has been shown from these experiments that the total energy estimated by Chittenden for some of the dietaries his subjects lived on was considerably less than the quantity necessary to meet the ordinary requirements of the body, and markedly lower than that essential for the body at work. The case of Mr. Fletcher, already briefly referred to, is most instructive from this standpoint. Professor Chittenden concluded that Mr. Fletcher was able to perform the work of a member of the Yale University crew on an intake of 1,700 calories. Exact observation on Mr. Fletcher for three days in the respiration calorimeter, most of his time being spent reclining very quietly on a cot, or sitting reading and occasionally writing on a typewriter, showed the average output of energy to be 1,896 calories, whereas the amount of energy actually derived from the food averaged only 1,357 calories.

In view of these results when at rest, Benedict states that it is safe to assume that Fletcher could not have taken the exercises of the Yale University crew on an expenditure of less than 3,000 calories. If the estimate of 1,700 calories of intake be correct, then he must have drawn on his tissues to an extent of 1,300 calories daily, or about one-third pound of body fat. Yet Chittenden records that not only was he in a condition of nitrogenous equilibrium, but that his body weight also remained practically unchanged.

How are these contradictory results to be explained ? It has been suggested that, while Fletcher oxidized his own tissues to obtain the extra energy required, owing to the amount of carbohydrates in his diet, retention of water took place, so that the body weight remained the same. This may be the true explanation, but it seems a strange coincidence that the weight of water retained should exactly balance the loss to the body through the disintegration and oxidation of its tissues. What appears a far more rational explanation would be that, owing to faulty methods, the caloric value of Fletcher's dietary during the six days was estimated at too low a figure.

This explanation is borne out by a consideration of the experimental work on Chittenden's second group of subjects—the members of the Hospital Corps. It will be readily recognized that a retention of water maintaining the body weight might act temporarily, but that it could not go on indefinitely.

What are the facts ?

Benedict and Carpenter* have shown, as a result of experiments in the respiration calorimeter on fifty-five men, with an average body weight of 64·5 kilos, awake and sitting quietly in a chair, that the average heat production was 97 calories per hour.

	Calories per Hour.
With seventeen men asleep, the heat production was	71
Man at rest, standing, the heat production was	114
Man at severe muscular exercise, the heat production was	653

Chittenden's soldier group led quite active lives, rising at 6.45 a.m., occupied with various duties all day, including two hours' activity in a gymnasium in addition to regular drills, walking, instruction in nursing duties, assisting in laboratory work, etc.

According to Chittenden's figures, the average heat value of the diet was—

	Calories.
From October to the middle of January	2,078
From middle of January to early in March	2,500
From early in March to early in April	2,840

The average caloric value of the dietaries for the six months of observation works out at a little over 2,300 daily. This amount, according to accurate determinations based on exact scientific experimental methods, would not be nearly sufficient to

* Benedict and Carpenter, "Metabolism and Energy Transformations of Healthy Man during Rest," 1910.

meet the demands for energy in the performance of the mildest forms of muscular activity, and, therefore, would be much less able to permit of the carrying out of the varied duties detailed for these soldiers.

Examination of the records for the professional and athletic groups would indicate that in these cases also the energy furnished by the dietaries, if correct, was insufficient to meet the different conditions that obtained.

The only conclusion to be drawn from these facts is that, unless all the world is wrong again, as Chittenden believes it to be with regard to the nitrogenous requirements of the body, in holding that the law of the conservation of energy obtains in the human organism, and that we must therefore fall back on the discarded theory of vitalism, there must be some unexplained source of fallacy in the figures given for the potential energy of the dietaries on which the three groups existed.

We believe this fallacy can be explained on the assumption that the factors made use of in calculating the energy of the foodstuffs were too low, and that the diets during the periods of nitrogen balance do not accurately represent the total food consumption in the long intervening periods. As already stated, we had arrived at a somewhat similar conclusion with regard to the level of nitrogenous metabolism exhibited by the subjects of the experiment.

Since this was written Loeser, in a paper* dealing with the good effects of an increased standard of protein metabolism on the stamina and general efficiency of miners in the Transvaal, states that inquiries, made from the soldiers of Chittenden's second group, elicited the important information that the men admit to have had "square meals on the quiet" during the whole period of the experiment. If this was really the case, it would explain much that is otherwise inexplicable in Chittenden's results, as discussed above, and would lessen considerably the value of his conclusions as regards the protein needs of the body.

Against the conclusions arrived at by Chittenden, we have cited a considerable number of facts and observations based on the known effects and results that follow existence on dietaries low in protein. We shall now turn to the evidence afforded by the inhabitants of large tracts of India, and consider what light the conditions that obtain throw on the merits or demerits of dietaries poor in protein.

* *Transvaal Med. Journ.*, 1912.

CHAPTER VII

THE EFFECTS OF A LOW PROTEIN DIETARY IN THE TROPICS

Effeminacy of the Inhabitants of Indostan.

"Southward of Lahore we see throughout India a race of men whose make, physiognomy, and muscular strength convey ideas of an effeminacy which surprises when pursued through such numbers of the species and when compared to the form of the European who is making the observation. The muscular strength of the Indian is still less than might be expected from the appearance of the texture of his frame. Two English sawyers have performed in one day the work of thirty-two Indians. The stature of the Indian is various: the northern inhabitant is as tall as the generality of our own nation; more to the south, the height diminishes rapidly, and on the coast of Coromandel we meet with many whose stature would appear dwarfish, if this idea were not taken off by the fineness and regularity of their figures. Brought into the world with a facility unknown to the labours of European women; never shackled in their infancy by ligatures; sleeping on their backs without pillows, they are in general very straight, and there are few deformed persons amongst them.

"Labour produces not the same effects on the human frame in Indostan as in other countries; the common people of all sorts are a diminutive race in comparison with those of higher castes and better fortunes. Nature seems to have showered beauty on the fairer sex throughout India with a more lavish hand than in most countries. They are all, without exception, fit to be married before thirteen, and wrinkled before thirty—flowers of too short duration not to be delicate and too delicate to last long.

"Montesquieu attributes much of the effects to climate, and

his critics impute to him to have attributed much more to this effect than he really does. It is certain that there is no climate in which we may not find the same effects produced in the human species, as in climates entirely different in situation and in every other circumstance. The Sybarites, whose territory was not more than a day's journey from the country of the Horatii, the Cincinnati, and the Scipios, were more effeminate than the subjects of Sardanapalus.

"To produce this effect of effeminacy in Indostan nothing is necessary but to give the man his daily food.

"The savage, by his chase and the perpetual war in which he lives with the elements, is enabled to devour almost raw the flesh of the animals he has killed. In more civilized nations the ploughman from his labour is able to digest in its coarsest preparation the wheat he has sown. Either of these foods would destroy the common inhabitant of Indostan as he exists at present; his food is rice.

"To provide this grain, we see a man of no muscular strength carrying a plough on his shoulders to the field. This slender instrument of his agriculture, yoked to a pair of diminutive oxen, is traced with scarce the impression of a furrow over the ground, which is afterwards sown. A grain obtained with so little labour has the property of being the most easily digestible of any preparation used for food, and is therefore the only proper one for such an effeminate race as I have described.

"There is wheat in India; it is produced only in the sharper regions, where rice will not so easily grow, and where the cultivator acquires a firmer fibre. All the Mohammedans of northern extraction prefer it to rice, as much as the Indian rejects a nourishment which he cannot digest even in its finest preparation.

"The Indian, incapable as he is of hard labour, breathing in the softest of climates, having so few real wants, and receiving even the luxuries of other nations with little labour from the fertility of their own soil, must become the most effeminate inhabitant of the globe; and this is the very point at which we now see him, A.D. 1753."*

"Their legislators have even ordained different kinds of food to the different tribes. The Brahmins touch nothing that has life: their food is milk, vegetables, and fruit. The soldiers are permitted to eat venison, mutton, and fish. The food of the

* R. Orme, "Historical Fragments of Hindustan," 1659.

labourers and mechanics varies according to their sects and profession.

"The Gentoos of the lower provinces are a slight-made people. Rice is their chief food. It seems to afford but poor nourishment, for strong, robust men are seldom seen amongst them. Though the people in general are healthy, they rarely attain to any great age, which is in some measure made up to them by early maturity."*

"Many of the Indians abstain from all kinds of animal food, and the greatest part of them use rice as their common and almost only sustenance. At the close of evening every man eats an inconceivable quantity of rice, and may take after it some kind of soporific drugs . . . the use of opium, which is to warm his blood for action and animate his soul with heroism. It must fill the mind of the European soldier at once with compassion and contempt to see a heap of these poor creatures, solely animated by a momentary intoxication, crowded into a breach, and both in their garb and impotent fury resembling a mob of fanatic women."†

The above extracts give some idea of the opinions of the earlier writers on the physique and the effects of diet on the Indian. It must be remembered, however, that in the period referred to the English had penetrated at no great distance from the coast, and had no knowledge of the splendid fighting material that was to be encountered later as English rule spread over the land. In order to correct the impression that the above picture applies to the people of India in general, one more extract must be given :

" I am afraid that the belief that the people throughout India live generally on rice is almost as prevalent in England as ever. There could be no more complete delusion. Rice, in the greater part of India, is a luxury of the comparatively rich. It is grown where the climate is hot and damp, or where there are ample means of irrigation. It is only in Lower Bengal, in parts of Madras and Bombay, in Burma, and in districts where the conditions of soil and climate are suitable to its abundant production, that it forms the ordinary food of the people, or enters to an important extent into the consumption of the poorer classes. Out of the whole of the population of India it is probable that not more than one-fourth live on rice.

* "Letters from Luke Scrafton, 1758." Bengal.
† "An Account of War in India v. the French on the Coast of Coromandel, from 1750 to 1760." Cambridge.

"Except in the rice-growing countries, millets form the chief foods of the population throughout almost the whole of India. Pulses of various kinds are largely consumed. Little or no meat is eaten by the poorer classes; meat is, however, commonly eaten by Mohammedans, and many of the Hindus who abstain from it do so because it is an expensive luxury rather than from religious scruples.

"The chief agricultural staples of Northern India are wheat and barley. They occupy nearly 60 per cent. of the whole food-producing area in the United Provinces. Wheat in the Punjab is a still more important crop than in the United Provinces. It is also extensively grown in parts of Central India, Northern Deccan, and Bombay, and in those countries, as well as in Northern India, it forms the chief articles of diet among the richer classes. Barley is largely consumed by those who cannot afford to eat wheat."*

In the preceding chapters it has been recognized that it is quite possible to maintain life, a certain degree of health, and a large measure of muscular strength, on dietaries whose protein content is considerably below the ordinary standards.

When it was discovered that the teeming millions of Bengal attained to a level of protein metabolism little more than one-third of that provided in Voit's standard, it appeared as if there was nothing more to be said on the subject, and that Chittenden's conclusions, based on the results of laboratory experiments, and carried out under somewhat artificial conditions, must be accepted as directly applicable to man under natural conditions and over the whole period of life.

This was freely admitted at the time, and it was pointed out that, so far as the knowledge derived from the analyses of the urine goes, it bears out in every detail all that Chittenden had contended for—viz., the feasibility of maintaining the body in a condition of nitrogenous equilibrium indefinitely on a diet whose protein value is one-third of that usually accepted as necessary for the needs of the system.

On turning, however, from a contemplation of the mere figures roughly representing the level of nitrogenous metabolism to a study of the people from whom the figures were obtained, other, and more important, points of view were forced on our attention.

* Strachey, "India, its Administration and Progress."

It was not, however, until evidence that appears absolutely convincing had been accumulated, that we unwillingly resigned our belief in Chittenden's deductions. His doctrine would be, for many reasons, a most comfortable belief to hold ; it is not necessary to enter into details of its numerous conveniences, but, from an official standpoint, it would be of immense importance to the State. In a country like India, where everything is on a huge scale, the economy in the feeding of prisoners, famine camps, plague camps, hospitals, and even armies in the field, with their crowds of followers, to be effected by the acceptance of Chittenden's standard would amount to very large sums, sufficient to fill the heart of any Chancellor of the Exchequer with delight.

It was, therefore, with many feelings of regret that we eventually turned from our original faith in the sufficiency of dietaries low in protein to become firm believers in a doctrine diametrically opposed.

When the average inhabitant of Bengal is dispassionately examined from the standpoint of physique, health, resistance to disease, and general manly characteristics, it became very evident that other things had to be considered besides a nitrogen balance and the mere fact of existence. What Hutchison terms " degrees of health," and Waller " the state ot nutrition," must not be lost sight of. The former author states that a survey of mankind will show that races which adopt dietaries deficient in protein are lacking in energy. " Energy, however, is not to be confused with muscular strength. A grass-fed cart-horse is strong ; a corn-fed hunter is energetic. Energy is a property of the nervous system, strength of the muscles. Muscles give us the power to work ; the nervous system gives us the initiative to start it.... If protein food, therefore, be regarded as a nervous food, a diet rich in it will make for intellectual capacity and bodily energy, and it is not without reason that the more energetic races of the world have been meat-eaters."

If this view is correct, then the Bengali, who lives largely on a vegetarian diet of poor protein value, should exhibit these characteristics to a marked degree. In the following pages we shall discuss the evidence on the ill-effects to be expected from existence on a low level of nitrogenous metabolism. Before doing so, however, it will be of interest to cite the opinions of some well-known authorities.

Macaulay: "Whatever the Bengali does he does languidly. His favourite pursuits are sedentary. He shrinks from bodily exertion, and, though voluble in dispute, and singularly pertinacious in the war of chicane, he seldom engages in a personal conflict, and scarcely ever enlists as a soldier. The physical organization of the Bengali is feeble even to effeminacy ... his limbs delicate, his movements languid. During many ages he has been trampled upon by men of bolder and more hardy breeds. His mind bears a singular analogy to his body. It is weak even to helplessness for purposes of manly resistance; but its suppleness and its tact move the children of sterner climates to admiration not unmingled with contempt. All those arts which are the natural defence of the weak are more familiar to this subtle race than to the Ionian of the time of Juvenal, or to the Jew of the dark ages."

Strachey, commenting on the above passage, says:

"There have been many changes since Macaulay's time, and among signs of increasing vigour one that is not without significance has been the development of a taste for athletic sports among the educated classes in the Government schools and colleges—cricket, hockey, and football, especially the latter, which is now played all over the province. This, however, is true of only a small section, and the general description remains much as Lord Macaulay presented it. It cannot, however, be applied to the northern and eastern districts, where the majority of the population is Mohammedan.

"The Mohammedan peasantry of the eastern portion of the province are men of far robuster character than the Bengalis of the western districts. It was among them that the sepoys who fought under Clive at Plassey were chiefly recruited, and the maritime districts supply thousands of intrepid boatmen and lascars to the mercantile marine."

There is no doubt at the present time of the fact that sport and manly exercises have taken a great hold of the Bengali youth, which may be accepted as a great step forward in the evolution of a more virile and energetic people. With this change in customs a demand for a more concentrated diet than rice is certain to arise.

The following saying concerning the Brahmins, who should be vegetarians, exemplifies the effects likely to accrue from foods deficient in protein:

"It is better to sit than to walk, to lie down than to sit, to sleep than to wake, and death is the best of all."

Bearing in mind that the great outstanding problem in nutrition is not the discovery of the minimum quantity of protein on which a man can live, but the determination of the level of nitrogenous interchange that is best for the efficiency, economy, and general welfare of the body, it has appeared probable to us that a survey of the food customs of the different races and tribes in India, living under as nearly as possible identical conditions, with careful observation of the effects on their respective development and character, would go a long way in settling the principal point at issue.

Such a survey we have made for the provinces of Bengal, Behar, United Provinces, and partially so for some of the people of the Punjab. We shall now take up the facts that have been obtained, and discuss the evidence afforded by these facts on the adequacy or inadequacy of low protein dietaries.

The Rice-Eating Bengali.

In Chapter IV., dealing with the protein metabolism of mankind, will be found a series of dietary studies carried out on some of the inhabitants of Bengal. From the information there furnished, the conclusion was arrived at that the average Bengali of the rice-eating areas lives on a dietary whose protein value is 55 grammes daily. This quantity was arrived at from practical experimental work on different classes of individuals, and from a careful collection of the average amount of foodstuffs consumed by large numbers of Bengalis. Full information will be found under the dietary studies referred to.

It was shown that the average amount of nitrogen excreted in the urine by the average Bengali was about 6 grammes per day. Making allowance for the nitrogen absorbed, but which is dissipated or disappears in other ways than in the urine, this would mean a low level of nitrogenous interchange, but higher than that indicated by the urinary nitrogen. However, for the sake of comparison and uniformity, we may adhere to Chittenden's method of computing the metabolism of nitrogen per kilo of body weight; the average Bengali will then show a nitrogenous interchange per unit of tissue practically identical with that stated by Chittenden to be sufficient to meet all the protein

requirements of the body—viz., 0·12 gramme of nitrogen. "These are perfectly trustworthy figures with a reasonable margin of safety, and carrying perfect assurance of really being more than sufficient to meet the true wants of the body, adequate to supply all physiological demands for reserve protein, and able to cope with the erratic requirements of personal idiosyncrasies."*
In dealing with the evidence of the effects of diets poor in protein, we shall make use of the memoirs already published on the subject.†

1. *The Evidence afforded by a Study of the Urine and Blood.*

Extensive observations were made on the chemical composition of the urine and blood of Bengalis. At first the question was taken up as a matter of urgent clinical importance to obtain reliable standards for the normal quantities of the different constituents, in order that rational deductions could be drawn when any gross departure from the normal was met with in pathological conditions.

Marked differences were obtained as compared with the standards given for Europeans in the ordinary textbooks.

The following tables show the results arrived at :

THE URINE.

Constituents.	European.	Bengali.
Quantity	1,440 c.c.	1,200 c.c.
Specific gravity	1020	1013
Urea	35 grms.	13 grms.
Total nitrogen	18 ,,	6 ,,
Freezing-point	−2·5° C.	−1·24° C.
Chlorides	15·00 grms.	10·000 grms.
Phosphates	3·50 ,,	0·918 ,,
Uric acid	0·75 ,,	0·452 ,,
Sulphates	2·50 ,,	1·880 ,,

Very decided differences were therefore found to exist between the urine of the Bengali and that of the European. The important of these are—The lower specific gravity, the very much less quantity of urea and of total nitrogen, and the higher freezing-point, owing to the smaller quantities of different salts.

* Chittenden, *loc. cit.*
† Scientific Memoirs, Government of India, Nos. 34, 37, and 48.

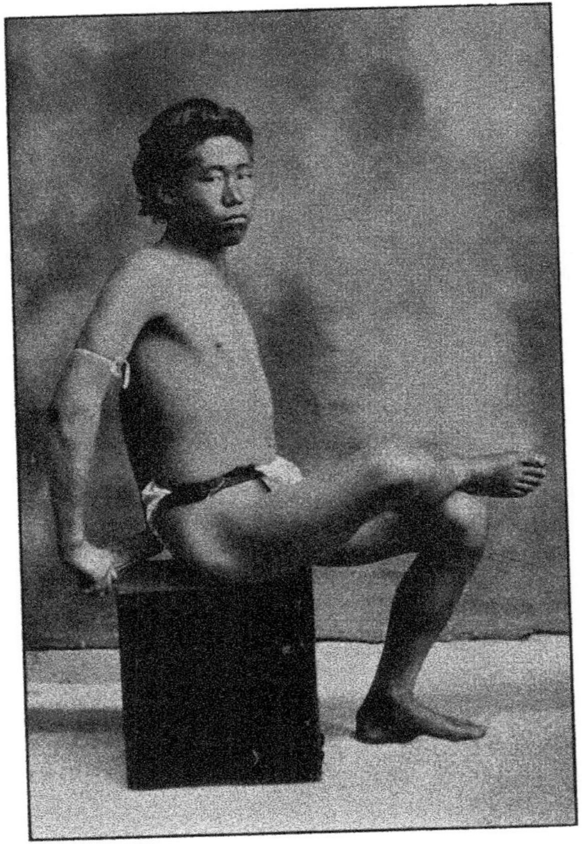

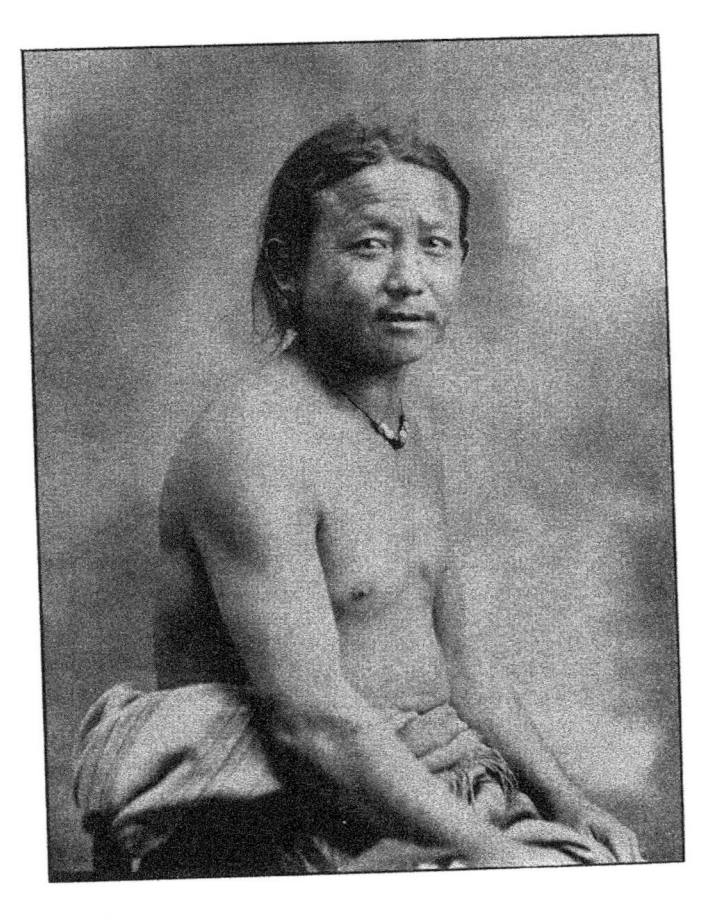

SIKHIM BHUTIAS.

THE BLOOD.

Constituents.	European.	Bengali.
Red blood-corpuscles	5,000,000	5,300,000
White corpuscles	6,000-8,000	9,000
Hæmoglobin	100 per cent.	81 per cent.
Specific gravity	1054-1057	1055-1058
Proteins	19·17 per cent.	18·23 per cent.
Total solids	21·13 ,,	20·12 ,,
Time of coagulation	4-7 minutes	1¾-2½ minutes
Systolic blood-pressure in brachial artery	115-130 mm. Hg	90-115 mm. Hg

[The figures given for the red and white corpuscles are slightly too high, as they include a number of observations made on some members of the hill-tribes.]

The most marked differences between the blood of the Bengali and the European are—The great deficiency in hæmoglobin, the smaller quantity of protein and total solids, and relatively, the much shorter time of coagulation.

A certain number of observations were also made on the alkalinity of the blood by Wright's titration method against diluted normal sulphuric acid solution; the alkalinity was found to be distinctly higher than in Europeans.

The comparatively low blood-pressure of the Bengali is of great interest from a clinical standpoint; it has been regarded as sufficient to explain the rarity of aneurism despite the marked prevalence of syphilis and its ravage, as seen in the wards of the hospitals.

From a survey of these results it will be evident that the Bengali is on a much lower plane of metabolism than the European. The standards fixed for the different constituents are of great importance in judging the degree of interchange of material going on within the body.

From our standpoint chief interest centres in the figures obtained for the urea and total nitrogen, and, as has been shown, these indicate a nitrogenous metabolism of about 0·12 gramme of nitrogen per kilo of body weight, using the urinary nitrogen as the criterion of protein interchange.

The condition of the blood is of equal interest.

It is evident from the analysis given that the protein content of the blood is deficient in the Bengali. This is all the more remarkable when it is recognized that the corpuscular element is quite up to the European standard. The percentage of the floating proteins of the plasma is therefore even lower than would appear from the figures. When we recollect that it is from these floating proteins that the different nitrogenous tissue of the body derive their nutrition, it will be abundantly apparent that these facts have a very important bearing on the sufficiency or otherwise of the diet, and more particularly of the protein element of the diet.

In this connection it is interesting to note that a sparing diet (1½ litres of milk daily) will cause a marked diminution in the amount of serum-albumin and serum-globulin in so short a time as one week.*

The blood-pressure has been found to be considerably lower in the Bengali than is the case in the European—a condition directly affecting the vigour and energy of the two races. The factors in the causation of this lower scale of blood-pressure are, probably, numerous. That difference in climatic conditions is not the chief cause is shown by the fact that Europeans living in the same climate do not exhibit such a low average blood-pressure as met with in the Bengali. As would be expected, the vasomotor system soon becomes acclimatized to the new conditions, and regains its function of maintaining the tonicity of the vessels in the area of peripheral resistance.

It is more than probable that the force of the heart-beat in the Bengali is less than in Europeans—the cardiac muscle, like the ordinary voluntary musculature, not being maintained in such a high state of nutrition as that permitted by the superior nutritive interchanges possible between the lymph and the muscle cells in the European.

The very great deficiency in the hæmoglobin value of the blood in the Bengali is noteworthy. From a large number of observations, both published and unpublished, the average amount of hæmoglobin is rarely found to exceed 80 per cent. This means that, instead of each red blood-cell being in possession of its normal amount of hæmoglobin, it contains, on the average, only about 75 per cent. of that quantity. This must have a serious deleterious influence on the oxygen-carrying capacity of the blood.

From the evidence afforded by the chemical composition of

* Landau, " Osmostischen Druck des Blutes."

the blood, it may fairly be deduced that the diet—poor in nitrogen —is the cause of the deficiencies. The blood in chronic underfeeding is said not to show, as a rule, any great variations in composition, being able to maintain its normal state under very adverse circumstances; but the changes that do occur are all of the same type as those discovered in the blood of the Bengali. V. Hoesslin states that chronic under-feeding influences the total volume of the blood, as well as the mass of all the tissues, and produces individuals who are poorly supplied with blood, fat, and muscle.

It may, therefore, be concluded from these analyses that the Bengali falls short of the European standards. His nitrogenous tissues are not given the option of drawing their nutritive material from so rich a source, nor have they the same opportunity of obtaining as free a supply of oxygen. The effects of these conditions must be to modify very markedly the physiological requirements of nutrition, and to a considerable extent affect the growth, power of muscular contraction, and general metabolism of the individuals of such a community.

While it is impossible to state dogmatically that these differences are entirely due to an insufficient supply of protein in the food, it would appear to be the most plausible, and, so far as the facts go, the only explanation.

We think we are justified in saying that a people who excrete only 6 grammes of nitrogen daily in the urine live in a chronic state of nitrogenous starvation, leading to a loss of body fat and tissue protein, with the inevitable result of loss of vigour and strength, and a comparatively low capacity for prolonged or sustained muscular effort.

Extracts from the older writers have been already given bearing on the working capacity of a rice-fed people, and we shall have further evidence to produce on this subject. At present it will be sufficient to state that the Bengali falls far short of the ordinary European in this respect.

This is not due to any deficiency in the energy-producing carbonaceous material, in which element their diet is very rich. We hold, on the other hand, that it is due to a lack of muscular development, and to the lower condition of vitality that must follow from the presence of a composition of the blood exhibiting the lower physiological limits of such necessary constituents as hæmoglobin and floating proteins of the plasma, combined with a lower scale of blood-pressure.

All these factors react not only on the muscular tissues, but affect every tissue of the body, and particularly the delicate mechanism of the central nervous system.

Mosso's work has taught us that fatigue is much more intimately associated with changes in the central nervous system than with mere fatigue of muscle substance, due either to accumulation of waste-products or the consumption of the reserve of energy-producing material.

It would therefore appear that, in a condition in which the metabolic chemical changes of the central nervous system are kept continually at a low level—as in the Bengali—fatigue will be more easily and readily produced. Such is indeed in accord with our everyday experience, and such we believe to be an important factor in the causation of the lack of energy and vigour which is a characteristic of the race.

2. *The Evidence afforded by a Study of the Physical Development of Bengali and Eurasian Students living under the Same Conditions, but on Different Dietaries.*

One of the large colleges in Calcutta kept a carefully tabulated record for over twenty years of certain data concerning each of its students—Bengali or Eurasian. The points observed were the age, weight, chest-girth, and height, which were noted every year for each student while he was a member of the institution. As a rule the students remained four years, but the data for the fourth year being defective, only three years are taken into consideration.

The dietaries partaken of by the two classes of students were also available. The Bengali and Eurasian lived under the same conditions, did the same work, and, as far as it is possible to have it, everything connected with the two classes was strictly comparable. The only difference between them may be summed up in two words—race and diet.

With regard to race, the term Eurasian in the present connection is meant to apply to all degrees of admixture from the pure native Christian to the practically pure white of European parentage. The great majority were considerably more native than European. As we have already pointed out, the average

Eurasian, unless properly fed, does not develop physically into a type much superior to the average Bengali. The conditions are, as a rule, very complex, many of the Eurasians of Calcutta being the descendants of mixed marriages between the Portuguese, French, and either native or Eurasian women. " Taking the native Christian and Eurasian population as a whole (though race cannot be invoked in the case of the former), the death-rate is almost invariably lower than that of the general native population. It is probable that the nature and variety of the food play a considerable part in the production of these results."*

The diets on which these two classes lived while in residence were as follows :

BENGALI STUDENTS.

Protein .. 67·11 grms.
Carbohydrates 548·73 ,, } Heat value, 3,100 calories,
Fat .. .. 71·55 ,,

about 9·3 grms., or 14 per cent., of the protein being of animal origin.

EURASIAN STUDENTS.

Protein .. 94·97 grms.
Carbohydrates 467·00 ,, } Heat value, 2,830 calories,
Fat .. .. 56·20 ,,

about 42 grms., or almost 40 per cent., of the protein being derived from an animal source, and more than half of the remaining quantity coming from wheat.

From the details, published in the memoir† recording these observations, it was shown that the Bengali students attain a level of protein metabolism corresponding to the interchange of 0·148 gramme nitrogen per kilo of body weight, while the Eurasian students showed 0·203 gramme nitrogen, undergoing metabolism for the same unit of tissue.

We have, therefore, two classes to contrast, represented by 568 Bengali and 126 Eurasian students, each class on a known diet, each entering college in their seventeenth or eighteenth year of age, living under exactly similar conditions as to the climate, surroundings, and work, and each kept under medical supervision during college life. The data obtained from year to year afford reliable information concerning the degree of physical development attained by the two classes.

This, in turn, will give us a trustworthy test of the adequacy or otherwise of the dietaries as a whole, and more particularly— the carbohydrate and fatty elements being admittedly sufficient

* " Imperial Gazetteer of India," vol. i.
† Scientific Memoirs, Government of India, No. 34, pp. 49 and 57.

—will afford direct evidence on the effects of a relatively low and medium level of protein interchange within the body.

What were the actual results? From the records we find—

Bengali Students.

1. There is an increase in the body weight, on an average over the whole series, of 2 pounds only, when the weight on entrance and weight at the end of the third year are compared.

2. On a comparison of the average weight on entrance and at the end of the third year, 42·8 per cent. of the students show a diminution in body weight; only 15·3 per cent. gained weight continuously during the three years.

3. On a comparison of weight on entrance and at the end of the second year, 55·8 per cent. of the students show a diminution of body weight.

4. The chest measurement practically remained stationary.

5. As would be expected from the age on entrance, the large majority—over 80 per cent.—of all students show an increase in height, ranging from 1½ to 2½ inches.

In the face of these results it can only be concluded that the metabolism of 0·148 gramme nitrogen per kilo of body weight was not sufficient to meet the nitrogenous needs of these Bengali students, and, in from 30 to 40 per cent. of the 568 students under observation, was insufficient to prevent a loss of formed tissue protein as the diminution in body weight would appear to mean. These results are in complete accord with the conclusion arrived at from a study of the blood, urine, and metabolism of the students and servants of the Medical College, Calcutta, in whom, on an average, a slightly lower level of nitrogenous metabolism was found to be present.

Eurasian Students.

1. The average body weight over the whole series is—for the first year, 116 pounds; second year, 123 pounds; third year, 130 pounds; and fourth year, 135 pounds. That is, compared with a maximum increase in body weight of 2 pounds in Bengali students, there is an increase of 14 pounds in Eurasian students over the same period.

2. On a comparison of weight on entrance and weight at the end of the third year, only 2 per cent. show a decrease, con-

trasted with a decrease of 42·8 per cent. in the case of the Bengali over a similar period.

Practically 100 per cent. gained weight continuously during the three years—a marked contrast to the 15·3 per cent. of Bengalis who showed a continuous gain.

3. Less than 4 per cent. show a diminution in body weight at the end of the second year, while 55·8 per cent. of the Bengali students lose weight during this period.

4. In the Bengali the average chest measurement does not alter, while the Eurasian students show the following averages: First year, $33\frac{1}{3}$ inches; second year, 34 inches; third year, $34\frac{3}{4}$ inches. This is a considerable increase for the period during which figures are available.

5. Growth in height is even more marked than in Bengali students, practically everyone gaining considerably in height.

The dietary of these Eurasian students provided a minimum metabolism of 0·203 gramme nitrogen per kilo of body weight, whilst the heat value and carbonaceous elements were very much lower than in the dietary of the Bengali students.

It is unnecessary to labour the comparison of the resulting condition of these two classes; the facts stated, gleaned from the medical officer's records, speak with no uncertain voice, and force the unbiassed mind to the conclusion that, while it is possible to live on quantities of protein much below that fixed almost universally at 100 grammes per day by the races and people who are of greatest importance, any marked decrease below this amount is likely to be accompanied with, and followed by, a train of circumstances that are neither to the welfare nor to the efficiency of the individual or the race.

The results obtained from a comparison of these two classes of students are most important in appraising the merits or demerits of diets low and relatively high in protein. It is not a comparison of the physical development of Bengalis and Eurasian, but a comparison of the two classes during a period of three years of their lives, which they passed under exactly similar conditions, the only difference being the quantity and quality of their food, and, particularly, the difference in the level of protein metabolism possible from their respective dietaries.

We consider these results prove conclusively that, with a diet poor in nitrogen, individuals are produced who are deficient in muscle, poorly supplied with blood, and who exhibit defective development; whilst with a liberal scale of protein intake results the opposite of these are the rule.

It would further appear, as has been frequently shown in feeding experiments on animals and in man, that general body growth, and, more particularly, growth of the nitrogenous tissues, increases *pari passu* with the degree of protein metabolism per kilo of body weight. Exactly where the line is to be drawn regarding the amount of protein essential in an ideal diet we are unable to say, but we hold that the above figures point undoubtedly to an increase in bodily vigour and development taking place up to a nitrogenous metabolism of 0·203 gramme per kilo of body weight. This would correspond to an interchange, for an average man of 75 kilos, of over 95 grammes protein daily, and would mean a gross intake of over 100 grammes albuminous material in the diet—70 per cent. more protein than Chittenden considers necessary.

3. *The Evidence afforded by a Study of the Physical Development and Endurance, Capacity for Work, and Expectation of Life in the Bengali.*

(a) *The Body Weight.*—From the records of over 2,500 observations on the weight of students, the average is just under 52 kilos.

Major Buchanan, I.M.S., made a very large number of weighments of prisoners in the Bengal gaols, from which he shows the average weight to be 110 to 112 pounds (50 to 51 kilos).

This is about 25 per cent. less than the average weight of the European. The Bengali is not sprung from an under-sized race; his stature and general build of body-frame compares very favourably with that of Europeans. On the other hand, the spareness and the deficient muscular development of the average worker form a striking contrast to the condition met with in the average European labourer. While it cannot be accepted that a high average body weight is the all-important criterion of physical fitness or power of resisting disease, other things being equal, it will be generally admitted that good muscular development is a desideratum in the efficiency and well-being of a people. In connection with this question, it has been pointed out that a close relationship exists between the physical and moral development of men; with a low physical standard we are apt to get recruits not only small, but unsteady, wanting in mental ballast as well as in muscular energy.

(b) *The Height.*—The average height of the adult male European, according to Quetelet's tables, is 5 feet 5 inches to 5 feet 6 inches.

The average height of Bengali students we found to be 5 feet $5\frac{1}{2}$ inches. Buchanan, from an analysis of his collection of 28,863 heights of prisoners, would place the average height slightly under the above figures—viz., about 5 feet 4 inches.

(c) *The Circumference of the Chest.*—The average chest-girth of our series of Bengali students works out to be just below the minimum for admission into the British Army—viz., 33 inches. It is, therefore, well below the average European standard.

Landois lays down a rule in judging good weight for height, that normally developed individuals weigh as many kilos as their length measures in centimetres, after subtracting the first metre. This works out very well for the average height and weight of Europeans—Europeans 168 centimetres in height should weigh 68 kilos. When we come, however, to apply the rule to Bengalis, whose average height may be taken at 5 feet 4 inches, or 162 centimetres, we find he falls far short of the proper standard.

(d) *Physical Endurance.*—It is difficult to obtain anything like fair comparative tests between the rice-eating Bengali and the European labourer, but anyone who has seen the ordinary Bengali at work will not require much in the way of statistical evidence to convince him of the marked superiority of the European. The same remark applies also, to a certain extent, to a contrast of the working capacity of the Bengali and the better-fed people of Behar, Eastern Bengal, United Provinces, and Punjab. The picture of the feebleness, laziness, lack of energy, and sleepiness of the working coolie could hardly be overdrawn. We have seen three labourers, with, of course, a *sirdar* or overseer, take eight days to loosen the surface of a drive to the depth of 2 inches; the total surface area of the drive was roughly 200 square yards. Any ordinary European labourer would have finished the work in a few hours. On watching them for a time, it was noticed that the three took turns to work, with long intervals, when they all sat or lay about, and after an hour or so of this, one would disappear for a sleep, to be followed later by the remaining two in turn; the overseer slept most of the time, making no attempt to keep them at their work.

(e) *Capacity for Work.*—The following table, modified from the report on factory labour in India, brings out clearly the relative productive capacity of the English and Indian worker:

	England.	India.
Operatives per 1,000 spindles	4·2	28
,, ,, looms	43	125
Annual out-turn of yarn per operative	7,736 lbs.	4,000 lbs.
Weekly out-turn of cloth per operative	767 yds.	240 yds.
Working hours per week	55½	80
,, ,, ,, year	2,775	4,120

Indian labour is lacking in continuous application, punctuality, energy, and regularity. Men have to be employed in India for work that women will do in England. The Indian workers have little skill or education, and consequently make much waste; their sense of discipline is imperfect; their attendance irregular; and they take long intervals for rest, smoking, etc. (Commercial Supplement of the *Times*).

The coal-mines of Europe and Bengal are perhaps the best comparative test of the capabilities of the two classes of workers. The conditions are all in favour of the Bengali; he cuts coal from thick seams, the mines are at no great depth, and a large proportion are worked with inclines, no shafts being necessary. The following figures give some idea of the output per man yearly:

```
America     ..  ..  ..  ..  589 tons (mining simple).
England     ..  ..  ..  ..  300   ,,
Germany     ..  ..  ..  ..  243   ,,
   ,,       ..  ..  ..  ..  600   ,,   (lignite quarries).
Bengal      ..  ..  ..  ..   80   ,,
```

The physical conditions are altogether in favour of the Bengali, and the result is an out-turn barely 27 per cent. of that of the European.

We might multiply instances of the inferior capabilities of the native workmen, but it is so well recognized by all who have had dealings with them that further evidence is unnecessary.

It may be accepted that the rice-eating Bengali on a diet

poor in nitrogen is incapable of performing a really hard day's work; the explanation can only be that the deficient nitrogenous intake does not permit of the development of the muscular tissue necessary for the carrying out of severe labour.

The carbohydrate element of the diet is present in abundance for the supply of the required energy, but the muscular tissue, essential for the dissipation of that energy in the form of work, is largely lacking.

(f) *Expectation of Life.*—The following table,* compiled by Mr. Hardy from census and local mortality statistics, may be taken to give an approximately accurate estimate of the expectation of life at different ages, with the corresponding English figures for comparison:

Age in Years.	India, 1881-1891. Males.	India, 1881-1891. Females.	England, 1881-1891. Males.	England, 1881-1891. Females.
0	24·6	25·5	43·7	47·2
5	37·1	36·1	52·7	54·9
10	35·5	34·4	49·0	51·1
15	32·3	31·7	44·5	46·5
20	29·2	29·3	40·3	42·4
25	26·3	27·0	36·3	38·5
35	21·1	22·4	28·9	31·2
45	16·5	17·9	22·1	24·0
55	12·2	13·2	15·7	17·2
65	8·2	8·7	10·3	11·3

Between fifteen and thirty-five years of age the probabilities are from 36 to 38 per cent. for males, and from 34 to 48 per cent. for females, less favourable in India; the difference at birth amounts to 79 and 85 per cent. respectively.

The mortality rates per 1,000 are also much higher in India than in European countries. In Bengal the "probable true normal rate" (1888-1891) was 44·8 per 1,000, and for India 39·6. For the same period in England and Wales the death-rate was 19·1.

It is interesting to note that the figures for Hindus and Mohammedans show that the death-rates, under similar conditions, are in favour of the latter. This is the more remarkable

* "Imperial Gazetteer of India," vol. i., p. 515.

as the Mussulmans, as a body, are often included in the poorer sections of the community. In the Native Army, during the five years 1895-1899, the mean death-rate of Hindus was 8·8 per 1,000, while that of the Mohammedans was only 3·6.

Also, the available records of mortality from plague afford testimony to the greater power of resistance which Mussulmans enjoy. As already stated, Eurasians and native Christians have invariably a lower death-rate than the general native population ; these results are ascribed by the author of the article as largely due to differences in the nature and variety of food.* The Mohammedans, Eurasians, and native Christians are all meat - eaters to a much greater extent than the Hindu, and animal food in almost any form raises the level of nitrogenous metabolism in a way even the best of cereals fails to do.

Further evidence of the inferiority of the Indian, and more particularly of the Bengali, as regards the expectation of life, is afforded by information collected from insurance companies.

The greatest precautions are taken in the selection of Indian lives ; even then, those accepted are rated up 33 per cent. higher than Europeans in Europe.

Compared with Europeans in India, some companies add five years to the Bengali's age—*i.e.*, a Bengali of thirty years pays the premium of a European of thirty-five years of age.

Some companies only accept Bengali lives when insured for a limited number of years ; the fewer, and therefore the higher the premiums, the more welcome the policy. An endowment policy is rarely granted which matures above the age of fifty to fifty-five years. The explanation of this condition is that policies beyond these ages were found not to pay, death occurring before sufficient premiums had been paid to cover the amount of the policy.

Mr. A. T. Winter, F.I.A., states : " The most eligible class of natives are assurable at the same rates as Europeans in India, provided their age at entry does not exceed forty."

An important paper on life insurance in India by Dr. Adrian Caddy† gives some information on the physique and general

---

* "Imperial Gazetteer of India," vol. i., p. 515.
† " Life Assurance in India," Life Assurance Medical Officers' Association.

health conditions of the classes who are able to afford such provision for the future. These classes are, of course, drawn from those who are in affluent circumstances, or who are in receipt of a steady income more than sufficient to cover the ordinary expenses of family life. As would be expected, they belong to the middle classes, who are above indigence, and the well-to-do people—that is, the very people who can afford to live on a liberal diet. We have given in Chapter IV., Dietary Study 3, some idea of the food of these classes, and reference to the facts will show that the diets are well supplied with assimilable protein—amongst the better classes, reaching the almost universal average of 100 grammes of protein in the daily food.

The facts supplied by Dr. Caddy's paper on over 6,000 cases personally examined, afford a good means of comparing the physical development of those who are properly fed with the average Bengali who lives on the lower limits of protein metabolism.

Dr. Caddy's results show that—

1. The average height of the assurable Bengali is practically identical with those of the poorest physique in England. "Notwithstanding this, the insured Bengali is always considered to be a select person among the whole race, the vast majority of natives in India being quite uninsurable owing to their poverty and illiteracy."

2. The average weight for height corresponds very closely to the European standard for Europeans in India, though considerably less than that for Europeans in Europe, as indicated by Robertson's or Hutchison's tables.

It follows from this that the bony frame of the assurable Bengali is only slightly lighter per unit of height than that of the European—a very different condition from that which obtains amongst the average working-classes of Bengal.

Thus, from data derived from over 30,000 weighments of Bengalis, the average weight was found to be 50¼ kilos, whilst the average height over a similar number of measurements was 5 feet 4 inches (prisoners) to 5 feet 5½ inches (students). That is, whilst the height approximates fairly closely to the stature of the poorer classes of Europeans, the average weight is 25 to 30 per cent. below the European or American standard.

3. Causes of rejection among Europeans and Bengalis :

Of 1,799 pure Europeans, 8 per cent. loaded and 6 per cent. declined = 14 per cent.
Of 335 India-born Europeans, 8·95 per cent. loaded and 11·94 per cent. declined = 20·89 per cent.
Of 317 Eurasians, 7·88 per cent. loaded and 15·45 per cent. declined = 23·33 per cent.
Of 3,483 Bengalis, 8·38 per cent. loaded and 16·53 per cent. declined = 24·91 per cent.

Cause of Loading or Rejection.	Europeans (1,799 Cases).	Bengalis (3,483 Cases).
Inferior physique	1·55 per cent.	5·36 per cent.
Obesity	2·11 ,,	5·34 ,,
Glycosuria	0·61 ,,	3·24 ,,
Albuminuria	1·22 ,,	1·98 ,,
Sundry diseases	3·39 ,,	4·96 ,,
Hydrocele	0·22 ,,	5·10 ,,

The value of these figures from our standpoint is not so much that they afford a basis of comparison of the Bengali with the European—the European in India is generally a selected individual who has been passed as medically fit before leaving England—their interest really lies in the comparative information they afford on the physique, resistance to disease, and general well-being of the classes of Bengalis who are able to provide themselves with a liberal protein dietary, as contrasted with the conditions that obtain in the great mass of the population living at the level of nitrogenous interchange which Chittenden so strongly advocates as the optimum.

Dr. Caddy's figures bear out in a remarkable manner the statement made by us years ago, that the average Eurasian, unless following European customs and ideas on diet, was physically very little superior to the vegetarian Bengali, so that, whatever initial superiority his share of European blood may have conferred on him, it becomes entirely lost as a result of existence on diets similar to the native inhabitants, diets which are generally deficient in assimilable protein. The effects of a rational diet supplying about the European standard of protein material were strikingly brought out in our analysis of the evidence afforded by the observations on the physique of Bengali and Eurasian students under Heading 2 of this chapter.

The same effects have been observed in the development shown by Anglo-Indian and Eurasian students in residence for

four or five years in another college in Calcutta. A full account*
has already been published; it is, therefore, unnecessary to
enter into details. The facts are : These students enter as
mere boys of up to sixteen years of age; during the four years
or so of residence they develop into strong, healthy men, quite
up to the average European standard in physique. Their
dietary permits of a metabolism of 0·196 gramme nitrogen per
kilo of body weight daily. Contrasted with their native fellow-
students who live on a much lower protein dietary, the account
already given of their marked success in the intercollegiate
athletic sports, and the fact that, although few in number
compared with the number of Bengali students, the college
team was almost entirely selected from them, make abundantly
obvious the determining influence of diet, and particularly protein on the growth and well-being of mankind. The two classes
enter college about the same age, live in the same climate and
under very similar conditions; further, as we pointed out some
years ago, and this has been corroborated by Dr. Caddy's figures,
there is no racial reason why the Bengali, if he were properly
fed, should not be as well developed and as efficient as the
Eurasian; the results, however, at the end of their college
career are very different.

We may conclude, therefore, that whether we compare the
average Bengali with the European, Eurasian, or with the
Bengali who obtains a fairly liberal allowance of protein;
whether we contrast students living under similar conditions, except those pertaining to diet; whether we study the physical development of the Bengali, his endurance, capacity for work, or
expectation of life—the results of observation and investigation
all point in the same direction. The evidence forces on us the
practical lesson that the generally accepted level of nitrogenous
interchange cannot be decreased to any appreciable extent
without damage to the growth, maintenance, and repair of the
protoplasmic tissues, and a lowering of the general efficiency and
well-being of the body.

4. *The Resisting Power to Disease and Infection.*

Chittenden holds that the smallest amount of food that will
serve to maintain bodily and mental vigour, keep up bodily
strength, and preserve the normal power of resistance to disease,

* Scientific Memoirs, Government of India, pp. 53 to 56.

is the ideal diet. This amount, he believes, is fully met by a daily metabolism equal to an exchange of 0·12 gramme nitrogen per kilo of body weight. Any excess beyond this amount imposes just so much of an unnecessary strain upon the organism, and more especially on the excretory organs, placing on them the needless burden of the elimination of an extra quantity of waste products, which is liable to endanger their integrity and possibly result in serious damage.

The important point, from our present standpoint, is the amount of food that "preserves the normal powers of resistance to disease." The Bengali exists on the actual amount of protein Chittenden declares to be the optimum, and should, therefore, exhibit those "many suggestions of improvement in bodily health, of greater efficiency in working power, and greater freedom from disease," which Chittenden believes to be amongst the merits of diets poor in protein.

It may be stated at once that there is absolutely no evidence to support the contention that the elimination of the waste products of the average protein dietary throws any strain on the kidneys—in fact, the evidence would tend to point to exactly the opposite conclusion—viz., that there is greater danger of a condition of malnutrition of the renal epithelium from the lowered or impoverished state of the blood which accompanies a diet poor in protein. In support of this view we may point out—

1. The great prevalence of kidney disease in Bengal, despite the very low level of nitrogenous interchange exhibited by the great mass of the population.

2. The very common association of albuminuria with the ordinary dietetic form of glycosuria found in Bengal, even in the earlier stages of the disease. Dr. Chuni Lal Bose* states that 65 per cent. of his series of 325 cases of glycosuria showed evidence of kidney damage. In Europeans glycosuria is not accompanied by albuminuria in anything like such a high percentage of cases. We believe that the explanation rests largely with the nutritive power of the plasma in the two classes of people, the lowered state of vitality of the renal epithelium, from the poor condition of the blood, rendering it more easily damaged in the Bengali, and less able to withstand the irritating effects of sugar elimination.

* Scientific Memoirs, Government of India, No. 34, pp. 63-67. This point is discussed in more detail.

NEPALESE COOLIES FROM NEPAL.

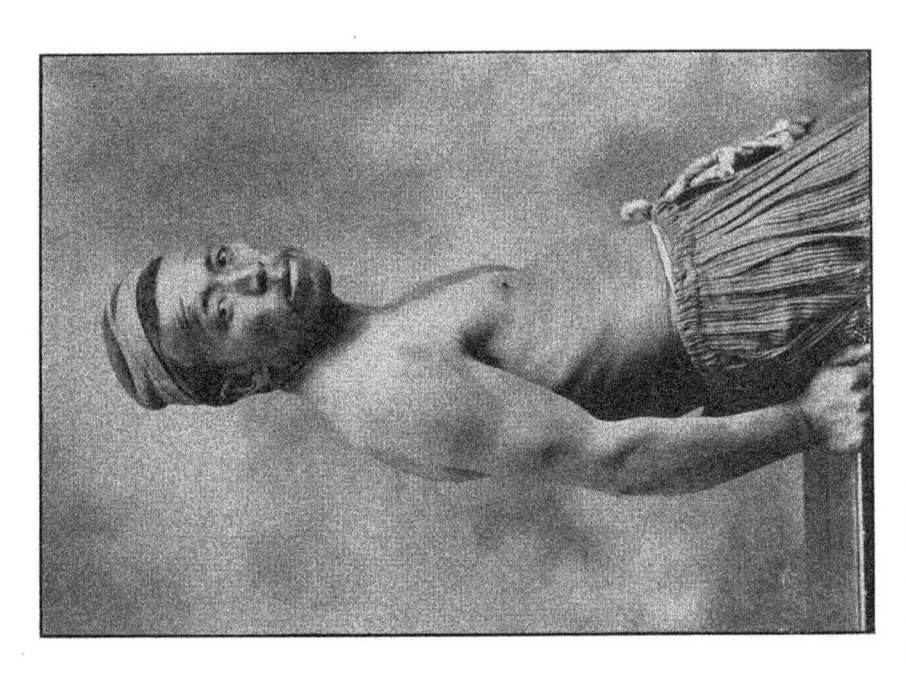

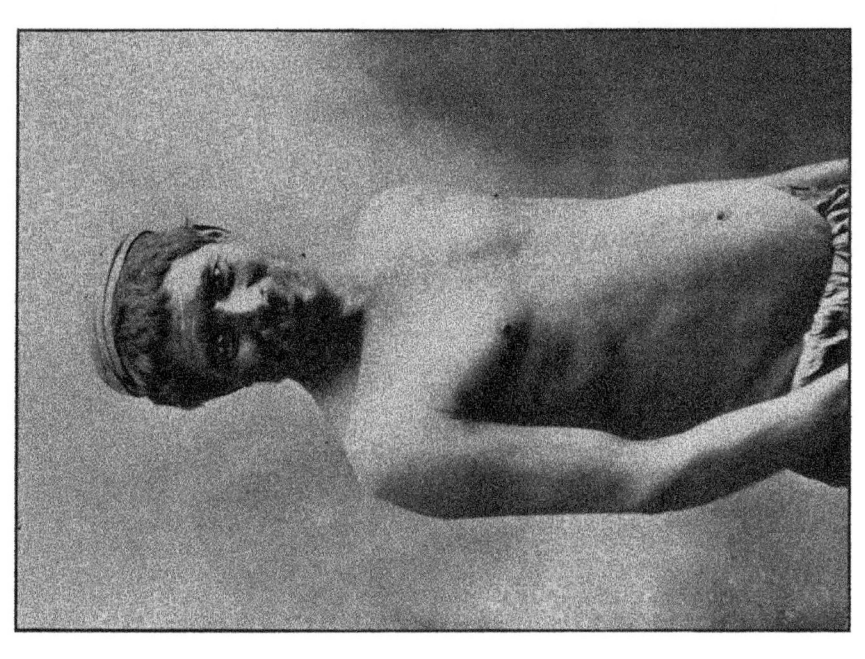

3. A similar common association of albuminuria with anæmia is met with in Bengal, in all probability due to degenerative changes in the kidney epithelium, from an impoverished condition of the blood. This also does not occur to anything like the same extent in the anæmias of Europeans. It would therefore appear that the resisting power of the renal cells is on a lower level in the rice-eating Bengali than in the better-fed races.

In order to obtain information on the effects of a low protein on the incidence of renal disease, we have been able to collect some valuable evidence. Thus—

Cases discharged or Dead from the Medical College Hospital, Calcutta, during Twenty-Two Months from June, 1905.	Total Kidney Cases discharged during the Same Period.	Percentage of Kidney Cases to Total treated.
Total, 3,602	120	3·33
Europeans, 1,320	26	1·97
Natives, 2,282	94	4·10
St. Thomas's Hospital, 1904: Total, 2,589	136	5·25
St. Bartholomew's Hospital, 1904: Total, 2,512	95	3·79

The most recent figures for the Medical College Hospital, including only medical cases of organic disease of the kidney, are—

Total Admissions for Three Years, 1909-1911.	Organic Disease of Kidneys.	Percentage of Kidney Cases to Total treated.
Europeans, 4,568	70	1·53
Natives, 10,343	244	2·36

We are indebted to Major Leonard Rogers, I.M.S., C.I.E.* for some most interesting figures obtained from an analysis of the post-mortem records of the Medical College Hospital, Calcutta. No. VI. of his series of papers deals with diseases of the kidney. He finds that in 4,800 bodies examined, serious renal disease was present in 4 per cent., and was the primary cause of death in over 3 per cent. of all cases. He states that renal disease is relatively a not very common cause of death, judging from the post-mortem records, although there appears to be no lack of cases in the wards. In a more minute analysis of 1,000 recent post-mortems, most of which were performed by himself, 6 per cent. showed well-marked disease of the kidneys, mostly con-

* "Gleanings from the Calcutta Post-Mortem Records," *Indian Medical Gazette*, 1909-1912.

tracted or granular in nature, whilst another 5 per cent. exhibited minor pathological changes.

The race incidence of renal disease, as demonstrated by these records, is of interest from the standpoint of the influence of diet. In 4,280 post-mortems the following results were obtained:

Race.	Parenchymatous Kidney.	Granular Kidney.	All Diseases.
Hindus	54·1 per cent.	65 per cent.	67·4 per cent.
Mohammedans	24·3 ,,	19 ,,	20·5 ,,
Europeans	16·2 ,,	15 ,,	8·2 ,,

These figures show that kidney disease as a cause of death is twice as great, in proportion to their numbers, amongst Europeans as amongst Hindus, the Mohammedan occupying an intermediate position. The Hindu dies considerably less often from parenchymatous nephritis than either the Mohammedan or European.

These results are at variance with those obtained from the hospital statistics on the incidence of renal disease as met with in the wards, and as found by Dr. Caddy in life insurance examination. The discrepancy is, at least in part, accounted for by the fact that the earlier records contained a large number of post-mortems on European sailors amongst whom, owing to extreme prevalence of syphilis, alcoholism, and scurvy, renal disease was very prone to occur. Accepting the figures, however, as worked out by Major Rogers, they undoubtedly point to renal disease being a more common cause of death amongst the meat-eating Europeans than amongst the largely vegetarian Hindus; so far as the deductions are valid, they would tend to support Chittenden's contention that the kidneys may suffer in conditions where a large amount of waste has to be continuously eliminated. With regard to this point Major Rogers states that the average age of death is much higher in the European than in either of the other races, and that naturally granular kidney would be present in a higher percentage of European deaths.

We may sum up the evidence from this standpoint by stating that in a country where scarlet fever is unknown, the prevalence of renal disease is amazing, and would not appear to support the view that with diets low in protein disease of the kidney is less likely to occur. Renal disease is very common in Bengal, and, as met with in the wards of the hospital and out-patient department, is distinctly more prevalent amongst the low protein-consuming Hindu than amongst the more highly fed European.

With regard to the power of resistance to other pathological conditions, as, for instance, septic infection, acute inflammatory processes, recovery from shock, etc., Rogers's researches supply information and evidence which have been hitherto entirely lacking. We stated in a former publication on this subject that there was a general consensus of opinion amongst medical men that natives stand acute infections such as pneumonia, plague, cholera, etc., badly. The evidence obtained from post-mortem records bear out this opinion in a remarkable manner.

Thus, the reports of 4,800 post-mortem examinations show—

1. That there are nearly twice as many Mohammedans over the age of fifty as Hindus, and almost three times as many Europeans. The figures are :

4,800 Post-mortems Show	Hindus.	Mohammedans.	Europeans.
Over 50 years of age ..	5·7 per cent.	10·4 per cent.	16·3 per cent.

This corroborates the evidence already adduced on the expectation of life for the different races, and shows that the low protein-consuming Hindu dies off earlier than the better-fed Mohammedan and European.

2. The race incidence of death from acute lung diseases, excluding tubercle, demonstrates that Hindus are very much more liable to die of acute inflammatory lung trouble than either Mohammedans or Europeans. Thus 74·6 per cent. of fatal lung diseases were in Hindus against 67·4 per cent. of that race in the total number of deaths. The Mohammedan deaths were only 1 per cent. below the normal, while that of Europeans was 3·4 per cent. against a normal rate of 8·2 per cent. of deaths. The figures are—

Race.	Deaths from all Diseases.	Deaths from Acute Lung Diseases.	Total Deaths.
Hindus	67·4 per cent.	74·6 per cent.	4,280, extending over a period of the last forty years.
Mohammedans ..	20·5 ,,	19·4 ,,	
Europeans ..	8·2 ,,	3·4 ,,	

Rogers states: "This marked difference in the incidence of lung diseases, extending over so many years, must be racial in character, and points to a lesser resisting power to these acute bacterial diseases of the largely vegetarian Hindu, as contrasted with their meat-eating Mohammedan brethren, while Europeans exhibit still greater resistance to these deadly affections."

3. Rogers has worked out the figures also for another acute bacterial infection—viz., acute meningitis. The records of 4,800 post-mortem examinations show that 75 per cent. of the fatal cases of acute meningitis occurred in Hindus, against 67·4 per cent. of that race in the total records, while only 17·5 per cent. were Mohammedans against 20·5 of that race; Europeans are again well below the normal. The figures are:

Race.	Deaths from Acute Meningitis.	Deaths, all Diseases.
Hindus	75·0 per cent.	67·4 per cent.
Mohammedans	17·5 ,,	20·5 ,,
Europeans	5·0 ,,	8·2 ,,

4. Cholera is distinctly more fatal in Hindus than in Mohammedans, and is less frequently the cause of death in Eurasians. Europeans, on the other hand, get a very much more severe type of the disease than either natives or Eurasians, and the mortality is proportionately high.

Rogers's analysis of these post-mortem records are of very great interest from the standpoint of the effects of diet on the resisting powers of the different races to bacterial infection. Space does not permit us to enter into further details; the general effect of the evidence is practically what would be expected from the differences in dietetic customs—viz., the Hindu exhibits a decidedly poor degree of resistance to infection in comparison with the higher protein-consuming races. This is particularly marked during the frequent outbreaks in India of acute epidemic diseases, such as plague, cholera, smallpox, different septic conditions, etc.

The Hindu suffers more from gall-stones, much more commonly from cirrhosis of the liver, and all acute inflammatory processes; on the other hand, owing to his low feeding and its accompanying deficiency in blood-pressure, he dies less often from aneurism and cerebral hæmorrhage than the meat-eating

Mohammedan and European. Bright's disease, which, according to Chittenden's views, should be practically non-existent in the Hindu in contrast to the Mohammedan or European, is exceedingly prevalent. Atheroma and granular kidney are practically as common in the Hindu as in the Mohammedan, the slight difference in the figures being completely explained by

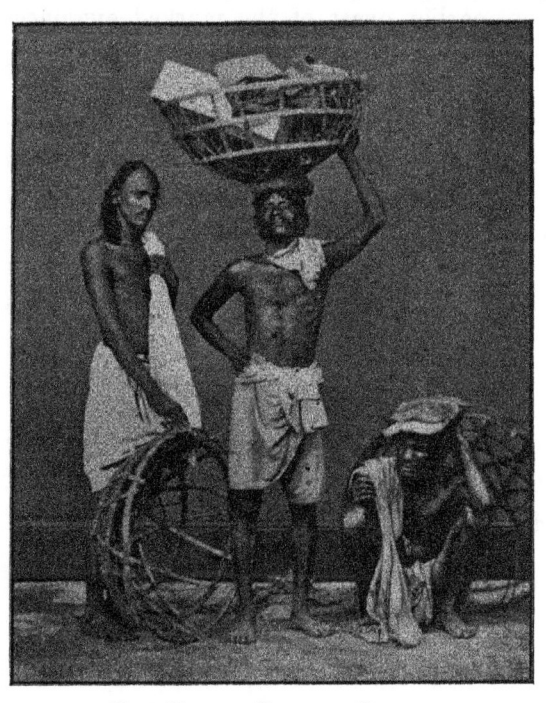

RICE-EATING BENGALI COOLIES.

the greater incidence of these conditions in the later decades of life, during which a much larger proportion of Mohammedans are alive. The figures show—

Race.	Deaths from Granular Kidney.	Deaths, all Diseases.
Hindus	65·0 per cent.	67·4 per cent.
Mohammedans..	19·0 ,,	20·5 ,,

NOTE.—Atheroma present : Hindus, 26·8 per cent. ; Mohammedans, 29·2 per cent.

Taking the total deaths after fifty years of age, the position is reversed—50 per cent. of Mohammedans show marked atheroma against over 52 per cent. of Hindus.

Such are some of the facts gleaned by Major Rogers from the post-mortem records of the Medical College Hospital, Calcutta. They bear out in a most remarkable manner the results of other lines of investigation on the ill-effects to be expected when a tribe or race subsists on the lower limits of protein interchange. The lessened expectation of life, decreased resistance to disease and infection, earlier onset of the marked evidences of tissue degeneration and senility, are conditions that would be anticipated in a people who exhibit such slackness, want of vigour, tonelessness, general slowness of reaction, and other physiological attributes difficult to describe, detect, and measure, which form some of the distinguishing characteristics of the working population of Bengal. Self-absorption, introspection, want of interest in the incidents of everyday life, little power of attention, observation, or concentration of thought—these are some of the attributes of all but the better classes and better fed of the Bengalis.

In the following chapter we shall take up some of the other tribes and races and study the influences of dietaries more liberal in protein on the physical development and general efficiency of their average representatives.

CHAPTER VIII

THE EFFECTS OF THE LEVEL OF PROTEIN METABOLISM ON THE PHYSIQUE AND GENERAL EFFICIENCY OF DIFFERENT TROPICAL TRIBES AND RACES

WE have now discussed the general effects of a low protein dietary, as exemplified by the Bengali, and showed that, from whatever point of view taken, the conclusion must be arrived at that his physique, capabilities of work, health, and resistance to disease, all suffer on account of his low level of protein metabolism. Before proceeding to an examination of the other tribes and races, it may be well to pause and ask ourselves the question: May there not be other factors beside the meagre protein interchange that must be taken into account before the condition of defective nutrition can be ascribed to the protein element of the Bengali's diet ?

Although our views on the relationship of food to physical development have been published for a number of years, so far only two serious attempts have been made to explain the acknowledged inferiority of the Bengali as due to causes other than those related to diet. One of these we have already referred to in Chapter IV. Chittenden believes the conditions met with in the Bengali are due to an ill-balanced, unphysiological character of his diet, and not to the limited amount of protein interchange possible from it. We have already discussed the misconception he was labouring under, and met his objections by simply pointing out that the average dietary of the great mass of the population is not of the ill-balanced type he considers it to be. The misconception evidently arose in his mind from our condemnation of the Bengal Gaol dietaries, which are in reality in no way representative of the diets of the people. We demonstrated, judging by his own standard of what a well-balanced diet should be, that the ordinary diet of the great bulk of the population does not compare unfavourably in the amount of unabsorbed protein with the diets by means of which he obtained his unique results. We need not refer further to this criticism, as it does not apply to the people whom we are discussing, and it really only holds good for the gaol dietaries, as pointed out by us at the time.

The second and more important criticism is that made by Dr. Kellogg. His objections have been of very great service to us, and have materially assisted in crystallizing our ideas as to the best means of obtaining irrefutable evidence on the adequacy or inadequacy of diets low in protein. Dr. Kellogg's words were : " The weakest part of the report* from my standpoint is the remarks which the investigator makes in relation to the defective nutrition resulting from the low protein dietary. I do not think it is at all fair to attribute the lack of endurance often seen among the Indians to the low protein diet. There are so many factors which certainly should be taken into consideration. Among these are their sexual excesses, the depressing effects of the very hot, damp climate in which they live, and which predisposes to lack of exercise, the injurious effects of excessive prolonged exposure to the actinic rays of the sun, the cause of debility to which Professor Woodruff of the United States Army has been calling attention with some considerable show of evidence. Still another factor of importance is the immature age at which these people usually marry. Many of the Indians, however, are strong and robust people. I understand that an Indian regiment made up entirely of natives is the finest lot of men in His Majesty's Service."

It will be readily admitted that, unless these points can be successfully met, there must remain a considerable degree of doubt as to how much of the ill-effects can be ascribed to the dietetic conditions, and how much to the disabilities enumerated by Kellogg.

We agree that the causes he advances have undoubtedly an influence in retarding growth and lowering the general standard of physique, and if there were no means of estimating their influences, it would be impossible to state that they were not quite sufficient to account for the poor physique of the Bengali. Considerations of space forbid us discussing these objections in the way we should like to do. A certain amount of information will be found on the subject in a memoir dealing with the gaol

* Scientific Memoirs, Government of India, No. 34.

dietaries of Bengal, and much valuable material on their influences has been collected in Risley's book, "The People of India," and in the first volume of the "Imperial Gazetteer of India." From the point of view of their effects on physical development it is unnecessary for us to attempt to measure and appraise their value for the following reason :

By contrasting the nutritive conditions of the different tribes and races—in which the several factors enumerated by Dr. Kellogg are common to all, the level of protein interchange forming the main point of difference—we can eliminate the influence of the sun's rays, early marriages, climate, sexual excesses, etc.—in fact, everything except the rôle played by diet—in the several factors that go to make one class superior to another, or one tribe or race superior in efficiency to another tribe or race.

In the following pages we shall, therefore, attempt to gain definite and precise information on the effects of diet *per se* by contrasting the developmental conditions obtaining amongst the people, tribes, and races who are in every respect, except with regard to diet, strictly comparable.

We have already given strong evidence of the determining effects of diet on different classes of Bengalis, subject to all the different causes advanced by Kellogg as fully accounting for poor physique. In this connection nothing could be more convincing than a comparison of the average weight, height, and chest measurement of the ordinary working population and the physical development of the better fed, assurable classes as evidenced by Dr. Caddy's records. Similar results were obtained from observations on students of the same and different colleges, living under similar conditions, but regarding whom the levels of protein interchange differed considerably. A full account of these observations will be found in the preceding chapters, so that it is unnecessary to do more than call attention to them in the present connection.

The rice-eating Bengali may be contrasted with his nearest neighbours, the people of Behar, as the conditions of life for these people are very similar. From work done on the protein metabolism of the Behari,[*] it was shown that the level of nitrogenous interchange is at least 20 per cent. higher than is the case in the Bengali. In accordance with this the Behari shows a much superior physical development, greater capabilities for muscular

[*] Scientific Memoirs, Government of India, No. 38, pp. 206-209.

exertion, and a distinctly greater degree of vivacity, tonicity, and energy. The body weight, and what is really of most importance, the actual quantity of protoplasmic tissue, is also on a higher scale of development. The evidence shows that the Behari is a stronger, healthier, and more capable individual in every respect than the Bengali, when the same classes of each, such as the working classes, are compared. The only explanation of this finding, from Dr. Kellogg's standpoint, would be the influence of climate. Behar is drier than Bengal, has a lower temperature in the cold season, but is much hotter in the summer.

The differences in climate, however, are only marked between the extremes of Bengal and Behar, whereas whenever we find a change from a diet of rice and dal to one containing wheat in addition, the superiority of the Behari at once becomes evident.

The same condition is met with in contrasting the rice-eating Bengali with those of the more eastern parts of the province, where fish forms an important element in the dietary. In this comparison even the influence of a slight difference in climate is eliminated, as the eastern districts are even more moist than those around Calcutta.

All the factors that Kellogg lays stress on are present in Behar, Lower Bengal, and Eastern Bengal, and yet it is well recognized that the Behari and native of Eastern Bengal is a much superior man physically to the inhabitant of the Presidency districts. The only explanation that will withstand the test of critical observation is that based on differences in diet. This difference is the substitution of a certain amount of wheat for rice in the case of the Behari, and of wheat and fish in the case of the people of Eastern Bengal, or—translated into its ultimate effects—the metabolism of from 8 to 9 grammes of nitrogen daily for the average Behari and Eastern Bengali, in place of a metabolism of from 6 to 7 grammes of nitrogen for the rice-eating inhabitant of Lower Bengal and Orissa.

It may be concluded, therefore, that, so far as the evidence obtained by contrasting the different classes of Bengalis, and Bengalis of the same race, but living in different districts and on different scales of nutrition, goes, diet and the level of protein interchange play the principal part in the formation of their respective characteristics, and is the principal factor in the building up and maintenance of the nitrogenous tissues of the body.

Before passing from the inhabitants of the plains of Bengal it is necessary to refer to the last part of Kellogg's criticism—viz., "Many of the Indians, however, are strong and robust people. I understand that an Indian regiment made up entirely of natives is the finest lot of men in His Majesty's Service." These remarks were made in connection with our work on the metabolism of the rice-eating Bengali, and their effect is to afford another example of the loose way in which evidence on the sufficiency of vegetarian diets is collected. The line of reasoning is easily followed : rice is the staple food of the Indian ; the physique and manly qualities of Indian regiments compare very favourably with that of other countries whose soldiers are accustomed to meat, and are high protein feeders ; therefore a vegetable diet and a low level of protein metabolism is quite as good, if not actually superior, to a mixed dietary and a higher level of nutrition. The true facts, as exemplified in the selection of soldiers for the Indian Army, demonstrate the fallacy of this reasoning, and afford still further evidence of the importance of a high standard of nutrition in the formation of the qualities and instincts of the soldier.

The Bengali has never, so far as we are aware, in modern times been recruited for the fighting line, and although many regiments are termed Bengal Infantry, Bengal Cavalry, etc., not a single man carrying a rifle could claim Bengal as his place of birth. We have no desire to labour this point unduly, but the question arises, Why is the Bengali unfit for the fighting line when other inhabitants of the great Gangetic Plain, stretching from the north-west in the Punjab to the sea in Bengal, exposed to, and suffering from, practically all the disabilities enumerated by Kellogg, but on a superior dietary, are capable of exhibiting the firmest courage, and maintaining untarnished the great fighting traditions of their race ? Thus, there is the Sikh, famous thoughout the world for his endurance and manly qualities, an inhabitant of the hottest plains of India, yet a man of splendid physique and full of energy ; the Dogra, the Jat, Rajput, all well known for their own special qualities on the Indian frontier, or where courage, determination and endurance are called for. Even in the various classes of these and allied races, differences in physique, muscular vigour, hardiness, and all those qualities that go to make up the perfect soldier, can be detected.

We believe that diet, and particularly the level of nitrogenous metabolism attained, has an immense influence on the formation of those desirable characteristics so well exemplified in the races whence is drawn our best fighting material. Further, although we have made little or no attempt to advance arguments for or against vegetarianism, it will be found that those races, whether of the hills or the plains, who are distinguished above all others for their martial qualities, are never vegetarians, but, on the contrary, usually large meat-eaters. The Sikh lives on wheat, other cereals, milk, and meat, particularly pork, of which he is specially fond. The Rajput, Pathan, Baluchi, etc., are all large meat-consumers, while the more or less purely vegetarian races, such as the Brahmins, are gradually being eliminated as recruiting sources for the Indian Army. We shall study the influence of the protein element of the dietaries of these races presently, simply pointing out now that the elimination of the several causes advanced by Kellogg, effected by comparison of tribes or races living under identical conditions as regards sexual excesses, climate, immature age of marriage, etc., brings out in its proper aspect the determining influence of diet on the character formation of a people. All the evidence we have been able to collect from observations on the different tribes and races of India points to a high level of protein interchange in the body being accompanied by a high development of physique and manly qualities; whilst under the opposite conditions, poor physique, and a cringing, effeminate disposition is all that can be expected.

The Hill-Tribes of Bengal.

We have given in Chapter IV. the dietaries of the more important and accessible of the tribes inhabiting the lower ranges of the Himalayas in Bengal. From a dietetic standpoint they may be divided into two great classes, each with two subclasses:

1. *Bhutias.*

(1) Tibetan Bhutias and Nepalese Bhutias.
(2) Sikkim Bhutias or Lepchas.

2. *Nepalese.*

(1) Chuttries—higher classes (Brahmins).
(2) Matwales (Mangar, Janidar).

These tribes inhabit hills whose height averages 5,000 to 6,000 feet above sea-level. The climate, though not so cold as that of England, is misty and wet during most of the summer months, and cold, bracing, and clear in the winter. The contrast between the Bengali and the people of these hills is very marked. They appear more like inhabitants of different parts of the universe, rather than neighbours separated by barely fifty miles of country. The men, women, and children are jolly, light-hearted, always laughing, joking, and chatting; the children playing, singing skipping as they run about, much in the same way as children do in England. This is all the very antithesis of what will be found in Bengal and Orissa. The children in Bengal are poor, miserable, pot-bellied little creatures, with little or no joy in their lives, compared with these happy-looking well-fed children of the hills. The hill people in general are very healthy, strong, and well-developed, some tribes being of really fine physique; they are full of energy, and capable of sustaining the most arduous labour and prolonged muscular exertion. The loads that even the women and little children are commonly seen to carry up the steepest hills are incredible, and could hardly be believed possible.

So far as the evidence goes, two factors account for the marked contrast between the Bengali and these hill-tribes—viz., climate and diet. The other causes advocated by Dr. Kellogg are even more in evidence, particularly sexual excesses, than in Bengal. Whilst there is no doubt climate has a great deal to do with the higher scale of general development and efficiency, that it is not the only, or even the most important, factor can be shown by a comparison of the several classes living under practically identical conditions, but with differences in dietary forming the one outstanding influence on their respective characteristics. The following facts were collected :

1. Bhutias (140 men examined).
    (a) Tibetan Bhutias.
        Height averaged between 5 feet 6 inches and 5 feet 7 inches.
        Tallest, 5 feet 9 inches.
        Shortest, 5 feet.
        Chest girth averaged between 35 and 37 inches.
            Greatest, 38 inches.
            Smallest, 32 inches.

The development of the neck and calf of the Bhutia is very marked for their height, an average of between 14 and 15 inches being obtained from the measurements

(b) Sikkim Bhutias, or Lepchas.
　　Height averaged between 5 feet 4 inches and 5 feet 6 inches.
　　　Tallest, 5 feet 7 inches.
　　　Shortest, 5 feet.
　　Chest girth, the same as in Tibetan Bhutias. (Pure Lepchas are slightly smaller in stature than this.)

2. Nepalese (64 men examined).
　　Height averaged between 5 feet 2 inches and 5 feet 4 inches.
　　　Tallest, 5 feet 6 inches.
　　　Shortest, 4 feet 8 inches.
　　Chest girth averaged between 32 and 34 inches.
　　　Greatest, 36 inches.
　　　Smallest, 30 inches.

The Tibetan Bhutias are probably the finest specimens of manhood amongst these hill-tribes. They are stronger physically and more powerfully developed than the Sikkimese or Nepalese. Most of the really hard work, such as carrying dandies, hauling rickshas, etc., is performed by these people. The women are equally well developed, and are capable of carrying out the most trying muscular ordeals; young girls will readily undertake the transport of the heaviest trunks and articles of baggage up the very steep paths in Darjeeling and its precincts. The Bhutia from his earliest years is accustomed to weight-carrying, the children being loaded with weights they can just stagger under. As years go on and strength improves, greater and heavier burdens are carried, until in adult life loads of 200 pounds and upwards are easily managed. A working coolie will go steadily on carrying such loads all day, making trip after trip in a way never met with in Bengal. The constancy of the Bhutia's working capacity is a most noticeable feature when contrasted with the methods of the Bengal coolie, who, after even the slightest exertion, must have a rest and, if possible, a sleep to recover from the consequent exhaustion.

Amongst the hill-tribes themselves the Nepalese and Tibetan Bhutias are the finest specimens of manhood in every respect; next to them come the Sikkim Bhutias, and then the Nepalese. It will be observed from the data collected that the Nepalese are considerably smaller in stature than the Bhutias. They are also less hardy and less muscular. The Nepalese are usually to be found as ordinary working coolies or as house servants —i.e., in situations requiring considerably less expenditure of energy than in the work performed by Bhutias. These tribes are all purely Mongoloid in type, there being little or no admixture of Indo-Aryan or Dravidian elements (Risley). Their customs (a.) TIBETAN WOMAN FROM GYANTZE. 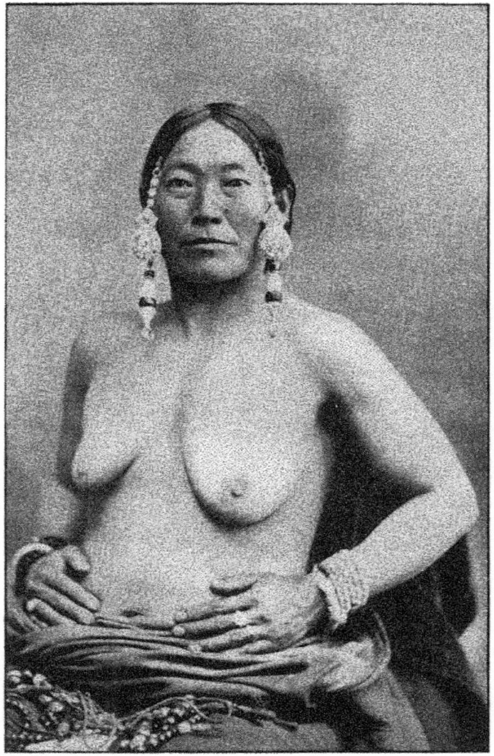 (b.) TIBETAN WOMAN FROM LHASSA. 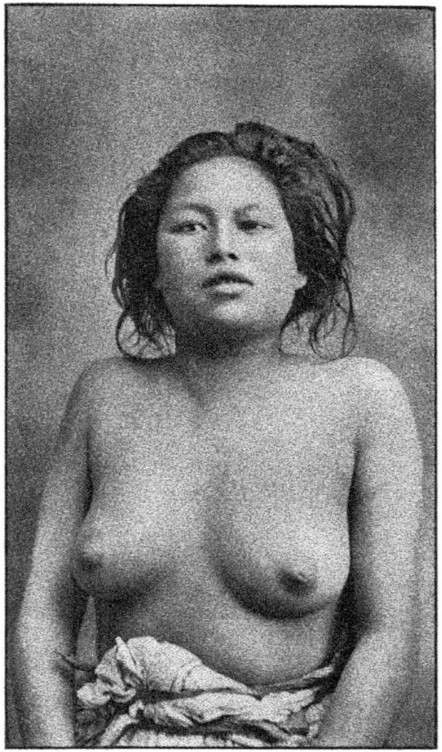 (c.) NEPALESE WOMAN.

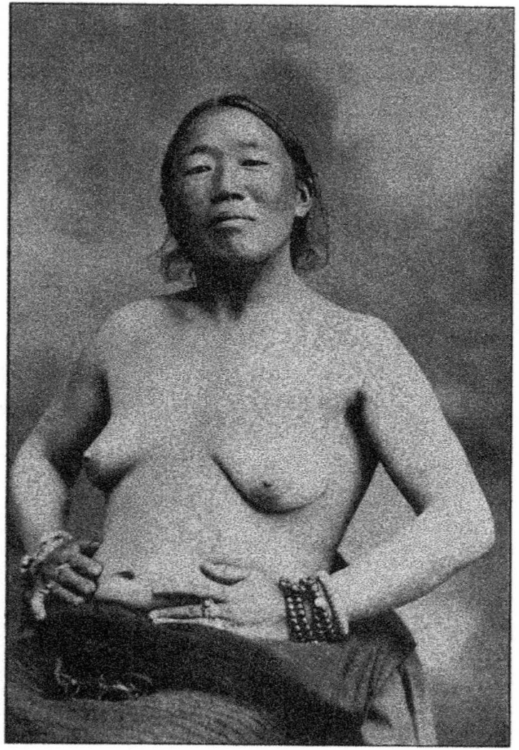

with regard to marriage, sexual matters, outdoor life, and exercise, are, so far as we could obtain evidence, practically identical, and yet within these tribes, derived from the same stock, living under similar climatic and tribal conditions, marked differences in physique have developed.

We hold that, while there may be other factors to account for the superiority of the Tibetan and Nepalese Bhutia, diet and the high level of protein metabolism he attains have a most important influence in determining his manly form and energetic disposition. We have given details already of the dietaries of the tribes inhabiting the hills of Bengal, and reference to them will show that the more nutritive the diet, and the more assimilable the protein element, the higher the tribe's place physically in the scale of mankind. From actual work* done on representatives of these tribes, it was found that the dietaries show a gradual decline in the amount of nitrogen per kilo of body weight undergoing metabolism, and in accordance with this there is an accompanying fall in the physique and general efficiency of the different tribes from Nepalese and Tibetan Bhutias to Sikkim Bhutias, and lastly to the lower classes of Nepalese.

This can only be explained on the basis of differences in diet; the other factors put forward by Kellogg are common to all the tribes. To anyone who has seen the powerful, muscular dandy-carriers of Darjeeling, and the much slighter though compactly built Nepalese, no evidence will be required to bring out the superior physical development of the former; and when along with this we find the Bhutia attaining a much higher level of protein interchange than the Nepalese, the conclusion that a close relationship exists between the scale of protein metabolism and the growth and development of the tissues of the body is justifiable. The average values of the dietaries of these hill people was found to be—

1. Tibetan Bhutias, Bhutias from Bhotan (dandy-carriers, ricksha-men, etc., who do the hardest work):
    Protein, 175 grms., of which over 60 per cent. is derived from animal source.
2. Sikkim Bhutias (hard-working classes):
    Protein, 131 grms., of which over 70 per cent. is derived from an animal source.
3. Nepalese Matwali (cultivators, coolies of poorer classes):
    Protein, 110 grms., of which only a small percentage is derived from an animal source.

---

* Scientific Memoirs, Government of India, No. 38.

188   THE PROTEIN ELEMENT IN NUTRITION

From a study of the hill-tribes around Darjeeling it is evident that the well-developed and more muscular races are those whose diet is very superior in the amount of absorbable protein it presents. The Bhutia, by far the most capable of these people in those occupations requiring great muscular exertion, attains a nitrogenous metabolism much higher than any other tribe. Just as was the case with the inhabitants of the plains of Bengal, Behar, and Orissa, so with the races in the hills, variations in the level of the average nitrogenous metabolism appear to be the determining factors of the several causes that go to relegate, fix, and maintain the position of a people, tribe, or race in the scale of mankind. The daily nitrogenous interchange of these hill-tribes works out to be—

1. Bhutias :   N per Kilo of Body Weight.
    Nepalese Bhutias   ..   ..   ..   0·42 grm. (very highly animal diet).
    Tibetan and Bhotan   ..   ..   ..   0·35 grm.
    Sikkim Bhutias   ..   ..   0·25 ,,
2. Nepalese   ..   ..   0·18 to 0·25 grm.

Contrasted with—

3. Beharis and Eastern Bengalis   ..   ..   0 14 to 0·16 grm.
4. Bengalis and Ooriyas (rice diet largely)   ..   0·116 to 0·12 grm.

The Races of the Gangetic Plain.

Of all factors other than diet that influence the stature and general physical endowment of the people of India, race or the particular stock from which the tribes originally sprung is of first importance.

Risley states that race differences play a larger part in the distribution of stature in India than is the case in Europe. The tallest statures are massed in Baluchistan, the Punjab, and Rajputana, and a progressive decline may be traced down the Valley of the Ganges.

In discussing the effects of diet as exhibited by the inhabitants of the Punjab, United Provinces, Behar, and Bengal, it is of importance to take into account the influence of race, and, by a comparison of tribes from the same stock, to eliminate this factor in the same manner as those laid stress on by Kellogg. This we have done in discussing the people of Bengal, who are all Mongolo-Dravidian in type—one of the most distinctive types in India. It occupies the delta of the Ganges and its tributaries, from the confines of Behar to the Bay of Bengal, and includes the bulk of the population of Orissa. In considering the effects of diet on the hill-tribes of Bengal, we limited the subject to tribes representing the pure Mongoloid type.

The only other physical types we are interested in at present are the Indo-Aryan and Aryo-Dravidian.

The Indo-Aryan occupies the Punjab, Rajputana, and Kashmir, having as its characteristic members the Rajputs, Khatris, and Jats. This type shows the highest stature recorded in India, ranging from 174·8 centimetres in the Rajput to 165·8 centimetres in the Arora. Individual measurements of Rajputs and Jats (Sikhs) rise to well over 6 feet. Within the Indo-Aryans, socially, "no gulf can be wider than that which divides the Rajputs of Udaipur and Mewar from the scavenging Chuhra of the Punjab. Physically the one is cast in much the same mould as the other, and the difference in mean height which the serrations disclose is no greater than might easily be accounted for by the fact that in respect of food, occupation, and habits of life, the Rajputs have for many generations enjoyed advantages, telling directly on the development of stature, which circumstances have denied to the Chuhra. Stature we know to be peculiarly sensitive to external influences of this kind."*

The Aryo-Dravidian type occupies the valleys of the Ganges and Jumna, and runs up into the lower levels of the Himalayas on the north, down to the southern extremity of Behar. The stature is on a lower scale than in the Indo-Aryan type, ranging from 166 centimetres in Brahmins to 159 centimetres in the Mushahar.

Although these physical types are largely limited to the areas given, it must be clearly understood that they melt into each other insensibly. The Rajput, for instance, is found in the Punjab, United Provinces, and Behar. From time immemorial in India a stream of movement has been setting from west to east, and from north to south—a tendency impelling the higher types towards the territories occupied by the lower.

As a general statement of fact it may be accepted that there is a gradual fall in stature, body weight, stamina, and efficiency from the north-west regions of the Punjab down the Gangetic Plain to the coast of Bengal; that this fall is more marked in a comparison of representatives of the three races inhabiting this

* Risley, "The People of India."

area—Indo-Aryan, Aryo-Dravidian, and Mongolo-Dravidian—but even amongst those of the same stock there is the same tendency to a lower form of physical endowment as the race is traced down the valleys of the Ganges and Jumna; that in accordance with this decline in manly characteristics it is of the utmost significance that there is an accompanying gradual fall in the nutritive value of the dietaries, and more especially in the average level of protein metabolism attained by the people of the Punjab, United Provinces, Behar, and Bengal.

In the Punjab the foodstuffs in common use are the better-class cereals, of which wheat is the most important. Besides these, different varieties of animal food enter largely into the dietaries of the great mass of the population. In the United Provinces wheat is not so much in general use, and animal food is decidedly less frequently consumed as a common article of diet; this falling off is continued as we get farther from the Punjab, until, in Behar, wheat is replaced to a considerable extent by rice, and in Bengal, rice is almost entirely used to the exclusion of wheat, except in the eastern districts. At the same time the animal content of the dietary becomes greatly diminished.

We shall now take into consideration the data available from observations on those tribes which supply recruits for the Indian Army. Accepting that the tribes recruited from are superior in physique, courage, boldness, and general manly vigour to the ordinary population, it will be readily admitted that it is of importance to ascertain the dietaries on which this superiority has been attained. If, for instance, it was found that some of our hardiest and best fighting races lived on dietaries of low protein content, we should have to acknowledge that such a finding militated strongly against the views we have set forth on the importance of a high level of protein metabolism; on the other hand, if with a high degree of physical development and martial qualities an accompanying high level of nutrition is found to be present, other factors being excluded, such a condition may be reasonably claimed as evidence in favour of the determining influence of diet on the manly characteristics of a people.

Rajputs.

Rajputs may be divided into two classes, Eastern and Western. The former are chiefly drawn from Cawnpore, Allahabad, Benares, and Lucknow districts, while the latter and better physical type of Rajput comes from Agra, Delhi, Rohtak, Hissar, Nabba, Patiala, and Gurgaon districts. Rajputs are the modern non-Brahminical and more or less pure-blooded representatives of the early Aryan immigrants into India. A great proportion of the Rajputs of the Punjab have been converted to Islam, and have therefore lost their distinctive characters as Rajputs. Some of the best Punjabi Mohammedans of the Indian Army are derived from converted Rajput tribes.

The two divisions differ somewhat in their caste rules and in their dietaries, the Western Rajput tending to be more elastic in his observance of caste obligations, and hence more amenable to changes of diet when necessary. The farther west a Rajput is, the less he is under Brahminical influence; the closer to Benares, the more priest-ridden, superstitious, and punctilious is he in regard to his religious customs. All Rajputs will eat flesh (except that specially forbidden), and do not object to the flesh of wild boar, though he will have nothing to do with the domestic pig.

Foodstuffs eaten by Rajputs—1. *Eastern Rajputs.*—Wheat and other cereals, juar, bajra, maize, and millets. Milk prepared in various ways, clarified butter or ghi. Legumens—gram dal, arhar, and urid dals. Little meat or animal food is consumed by the Eastern Rajput.

2. *Western Rajputs.*—In addition to those enumerated, animal food enters much more largely into the diet. Goat's-flesh, mutton, chickens, fish, and eggs are all made use of by the Western Rajput. Roughly, 75 per cent. of this class partake of meat regularly.

The dieting of the Western Rajput is therefore decidedly superior in assimilable protein to that of the Eastern Rajput, as the effect of even a small amount of animal food daily makes a considerable difference in the level of nitrogenous metabolism. It is significant in connection with this that the Western Rajput is considered so superior in those qualities essential in a soldier that the eastern branch of the race supplies a gradually decreasing number of recruits; some Rajput regiments have discontinued accepting members of the eastern branch entirely.

There is no doubt the Western Rajputs make far better soldiers than the Eastern. One reason given is that the former are far more pure-blooded than the latter; on the other hand, the differences in diet and in the consumption of animal food by the two classes is probably a far more important determining factor. There is abundant evidence of the truth of this statement in the respective physical conditions of different sects of Rajputs, pure-blooded or not as the case may be, when living on different dietaries. Thus the Rajputs of Jessulmer are physically much inferior to the Rahtore Rajputs of Bikaner and Marwar, although both are of pure blood; the difference is due to the fertility of the soil and the food materials available in the districts mentioned. Jessulmer is a comparatively poor country, and is incapable of producing wheat; bajra, barley, and gram are raised, but the higher cereals have to be imported. The effect of this is to lower the average level of nutrition of the population, and with this is found a lesser degree of physical endowment and a poorer martial reputation. The soil of Bikaner and Marwar, on the other hand, is good and fertile, producing wheat, bajra, rice, and other cereals; cattle, sheep, goats, elk, deer, etc., are found in abundance.

The same influence can be traced in those tribes of the Rajput race that have been converted to Mohammedanism. Thus the Sials are Rajput Mohammedans, who were converted to Islam in the fourteenth century. They are a fine type of men, brave, self-respecting, and hardy, with considerable pride of race. Physically they are big and strong, rather rude and rough in their manners. They are pastoral by instinct, but also engage in agriculture.

The Tiwanas, Gondals, Chibbs, Kharrals, Bhattis, are all of Rajput stock. These tribes offer splendid material for those regiments that enlist Punjabi Mohammedans.

The Rajputs of the eastern portion of the United Provinces and of Behar illustrate markedly the influence of diet. Priestly influence from proximity to Benares and a decrease in the amount of animal protein, accompanied in Behar by a substitution of a considerable amount of rice for the wheat of the diet, are the causes that explain the lowered standard of physique, and the loss of that pride of blood and race, and decrease in that spirit of self-reliance which so largely constitutes the martial instinct. The Rajputs of Oudh are being gradually dropped as a race for the supply of recruits, while the Rajputs of Behar have long since been rejected as unsuitable.

Physical Development.—Generally speaking, the physique of the Rajput is good. The Western Rajput is tall, well-made, with a good development of muscle, but somewhat light in bone. He delights in deeds displaying strength and courage, and is the most manly of all Hindu races. The following are the averages supplied by regimental medical officers for the physical development:

Height	67 to 68 inches.
Chest girth	34 to 37·5 inches.
Weight	147 to 154 lbs.

The Eastern Rajput is not nearly so well developed; the average height is less, and the body weight rarely exceeds an average of 120 to 125 pounds.

Dogras.

The Dogras are a Rajput race of Highlanders, preponderatingly Hindu by religion. Their country is most fertile, yielding large quantities of the various cereals and fruits. The hills abound in cattle of good breed, and agriculture is carried on with intelligence and care, producing large crops.

The following information is derived almost entirely from official handbooks on the Dogras, published for the guidance of recruiting officers in the selection of good fighting material. Written from an entirely different standpoint to that of this volume, it is of great interest to examine the views expressed by the authors* on the effects of diet:

The dawn of Indian history discloses two races struggling for the soil. One was a fair-complexioned Sanskrit-speaking people of Aryan lineage; the other a dark-skinned race of lower type, the original inhabitants of the land. The earliest records of the Aryans are contained in the Vedas, a series of hymns composed in the Sanskrit language from the tenth to fifth century B.C.

As the Aryan colonist spread, subduing the aboriginal tribes, there gradually arose four classes:

1. A class of priests—Brahmins—who looked after religious teaching and duties connected therewith.

* Colonel Bingley, Major Longden, Bonarjee.

2. As the simple life became more complex, a class came into existence who, relieved of the burden of agriculture, attended on the Maharaja; this warrior class was called Kshatriyas, and eventually Rajputs.

3. A class of agriculturists, traders, mechanics, etc., became differentiated off. These were called Vaisiya.

4. Lastly, the Sudra, or menial class, was composed of aborigines, and the progeny of marriages between Aryans and inferior castes, all of whom were excluded from the higher classes.

In course of time these occupational distinctions developed into separate castes, and as intermarriage became first of all restricted, and afterwards prohibited, each caste devoted itself more strictly to its own hereditary employment.

Prior to the Mohammedan conquest, the whole of Northern India was ruled by Rajput Princes. Some of these were driven into the hills and upper valleys of the Chenab, Ravi, and Sutlej. These hill Rajputs form at the present time the Dogras. They have been in these regions for over 1,500 years, have been largely untouched by Islam, and have retained their religion and caste rules almost unsullied during all these ages.

At the present time the highest class of Dogras are the Mians, who must never touch a plough. In earlier and troubled times this vow was easily adhered to, as the Mians were able to enjoy, either as a right or by force, the fruits of the labour of the shepherd and ploughman. In peaceful times this was no longer possible, and large numbers were compelled to take to agriculture. The Mians are those who have kept their blood unsullied, and their hands from the plough.

The Mians and higher classes of Rajputs, with the exception, perhaps, of the Jews, of all races in the world, are of the most ancient lineage and of purest descent. Though now nearly all agriculturists, Dogras form a military aristocracy of a feudal type. They are brave, chivalrous, keenly sensitive to an affront, and specially jealous of the honour of their women.

In disposition they are manly, simple, and honest, and, with the exception perhaps of the Dogra Brahmins, are little given to intrigue. The chief characteristic of the higher classes is pride of blood. It is among the Dogra Mians and Rajputs that we find the best specimens of Hindu character. We acquire a clearer conception of their high spirit when roused, their enthusi-

(a.) PUNJABI MAHOMEDAN.

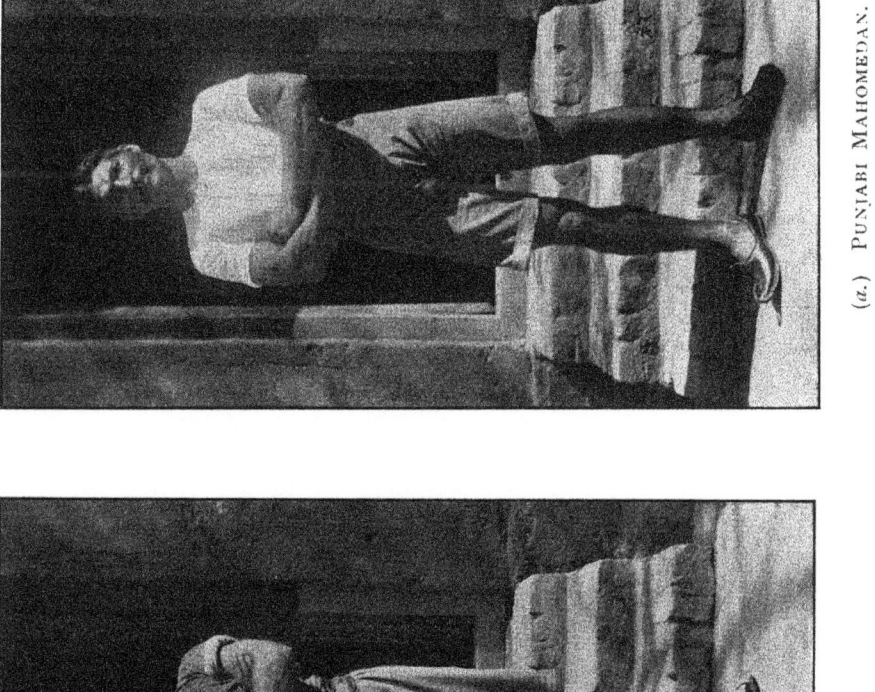

(b.) DOGRA.

astic courage and generous self-devotion, so singularly combined with gentleness and an almost childish simplicity of character. In no part of the world has the devotion of soldiers to their immediate chiefs been more remarkable than among the Dogras. They have ever been distinguished for their military fidelity and loyalty.

In vigour and manly strength the Dogra is not the equal of the Sikh or Jat. In their own country the Mians and Rajputs are generally inclined to be delicate. This is due partly to poverty and under-feeding from their dislike to agriculture, and partly to the prevalence of fever. When enlisted, however, they rapidly develop and fill out; but though good food, combined with drill and gymnastics, make them steady and well set-up, they rarely run to any great height, their average stature being $5\frac{1}{2}$ feet. The taller men amongst them are chiefly agriculturists from the plains, who, though physically more stalwart, have not the pluck and activity of the hardy hillmen.

Since the British occupation of Kangra, the Dogras of that neighbourhood have been compelled by poverty to resort to agriculture, though the highest classes still hold aloof from ploughing.

At the present time fully 70 per cent. of the population are agriculturists. In Jummoo, on the other hand, the predominance of the cultivator is less striking; here the Mians live in pride, poverty, and indolence. This acts unfavourably on their physique, which cannot be compared with that of the better-fed agriculturists of Kangra. Opinions differ as to the relative value of Jummoo and Kangra Dogras as soldiers. Both are equally courageous, but the Kangra Dogras are generally esteemed to be the better. They are said to have more heart, greater capacity for endurance, and greater pride of race.

The agricultural classes have usually three meals a day. Before going to work the men partake of bread reserved from the previous night's supper. At noon is eaten the first full meal, consisting of rice, dal, and bread made of wheat or maize. Supper mainly consists of wheat bread, rice seldom appearing. The different millets are largely used as food. Maize is a very favourite grain, and from September to May is in constant consumption. After May wheat matures, and for the remaining six months of the year wheat meal is the staple foodstuff.

Milk, curds, buttermilk, whey, and other preparations form a very important element of their dietary. In the agricultural districts milk and milky foods are cheap and easily procured; the effect is that the Jats, Sikhs, and agricultural Dogras consume large quantities, raising very materially the protein and nutritive value of their dietaries.

Meat is a luxury with the bulk of the people; they prefer goat to sheep. In most parts there is a good supply of fish, which generally forms a large constituent of their diet.

The strictest sects do not, but many Dogras do, eat fowls and eggs. Being keen sportsmen, they supplement the animal protein of their dietary with the flesh of different kinds of game.

As the great majority of Dogras are Siva and Devi worshippers, they are allowed to eat meat, a privilege denied to the worshippers of Vishnu.

In social and religious customs and practices the Dogras are very much like other Hindu communities, except that they are more superstitious and priest-ridden than the men of the plains. Infant marriages are customary, the only exception being in the case of the highest caste girls, for whom it is difficult to find suitable husbands.

We shall now give a few extracts bearing on the effects of diet as exemplified in the different Dogra sects.

Tho Dogra Brahmin.—In appearance the cultivating Rajput Brahmin can hardly be distinguished from Rajputs, except that their physique is generally superior, the result probably of the better nourishment they get. They make good soldiers despite their prejudices and indolence. The average standard of physique among them is good, and they are superior physically to the Rajput Dogra, as the Brahmin contrives to get more of the loaves and fishes of life than his co-religionist. They are notoriously given to intrigue, and are not really military by instinct, so that there is no great demand for them as soldiers.

Dogra Rajputs—1. *Mian Rajputs.*—This class maintains a most inveterate prejudice against touching the plough and against agricultural pursuits.

The adoption of agriculture makes a great difference in the physique of the Dogra Rajput. With more and better food he becomes more robust, and his muscles become more fully developed. The Mians, who still keep up their prejudices, are often thin and weakly looking, though a few months of good food and steady drill will work a wonderful change in their appearance.

2. The Rana and Thakur classes of Dogra Rajputs, with whom Mians intermarry, consist chiefly of the descendants of Rajput families which from time immemorial have been agriculturists. These classes are *par excellence* the most soldierly of all Dogras, and are of fine physique.

3. *Rajputs of the Plains.*—The Rajputs of the plains have lost the high-bred looks of their hill brethren. This is due to the fact that they have for centuries followed the plough. But agriculture, though unfavourable to their good looks, has proved decidedly beneficial to their physique, and these Rajputs of the plains are generally more muscular than the true Dogras of the hills. They are not quite so smart on their feet as the latter, but they nevertheless make good soldiers, and are generally very expert wrestlers.

4. *Lower Classes of Dogras.*—These are Rajput by origin, but have lost their social position. They are excellent agriculturists, steady, industrious, and plodding. Hence they are far better off than the Mians. They are of better physique, and have more robust constitutions than the higher Rajputs, but are not so refined. In military qualities they differ but little from Rajputs, with whom they are mixed up indiscriminately in all Dogra companies.

A good deal of valuable information on the influence of food is afforded by the above extracts from handbooks written by officers who have had long and close relationship with the classes discussed. The most important findings from our standpoint are the changes that have taken place in the physique and stamina of the Mian Dogras during the last century, despite their pure extraction from Rajput Princes, and despite the benefits of a hilly climate; the Rajput Dogras of the plains, and even the lower classes of Dogras of mixed extraction, on the other hand, exhibit in a marked manner the beneficial effects of good food on the virility and general efficiency of the individuals of the race. This influence is all the more in evidence when it is remembered that the great majority of these agriculturists and peasant farmers inhabit the plains and lower valleys of the submontane regions, where climatic conditions are not so favourable as in the hills, and where malaria is exceedingly prevalent. Despite these disadvantages, the well-fed agriculturist, both of the hills and the plains, has maintained his physique, the development of the lower classes of mixed descent improving under the favouring influence of good food to be equal to that of the pure-blooded cultivator; whilst the higher Mian Dogras, with climatic conditions and descent in their favour, but living on poorer dietaries, have within the last century gradually descended to a lower level of physical endowment, accompanied by a decrease in stamina, endurance, and resistance to disease. The Mians are the representatives of the great warrior class, Kshatriyas, who, in the times prior to British occupation, were accustomed to live on the fat of the land, and levied toll on all and sundry. For years they provided the very best material for the Indian regiments; now the peasants and even lower-class agriculturists are more and more largely recruited from; the Mians, owing to a lack of physique, being selected in gradually diminishing numbers.

Of the Dogras as soldiers, it has been said that they are not remarkable for daring or impetuous bravery, but they can always be depended on for quiet, unflinching courage, patient endurance of fatigue, and orderly obedient habits. They have not the grit and "go" of the better classes of Sikh, Pathan, and Gurkha; their soldierly qualities are essentially more solid than brilliant. Their steady, resolute courage makes them reliable, and they justly enjoy the reputation of being amongst the best fighting material in the Indian Army.

In physique they are not tall and muscular men, like the Pathan and Sikh, nor have they the physical vigour and sturdiness of the Gurkha. They are somewhat slightly built, of average height, with refined and finely cut features, fair complexions, and well-proportioned figures. Dogra recruits, however, caught young, while there is yet time for their physical development to take place, soon fill out with liberal feeding, drill, and systematic exercises. The general appearance of a Dogra regiment leaves nothing to be desired. The following data concerning Dogras has been supplied from a Dogra regiment:

FOODSTUFFS CONSUMED (AVERAGE PER MAN DAILY).

		Protein Value.
Wheat	12 to 16 ozs.	
Rice	8 to 10 ,,	120 to 135 grms., of which 40 per cent. is derived from an animal source.
Dal	2 ,,	
Milk	16 ,,	
Meat	4 to 6 ,,	
Vegetables	4 ,,	

The Dogra recruit, therefore, is provided with a very substantial daily ration, with very gratifying results so far as his muscular and physical development is concerned.

Average weight of recruits after six months' service .. 130 lbs.
,, chest girth of recruits after six months' service 33½ to 36 in.
,, height of recruits after six months' service .. 5 ft. 6 in. to 5 ft. 8 in.

The chest girth increases on an average ½ inch during the first six months in military employ—measurement taking at the end of complete expiration and arms extended above the head.

Jats.

The Jats also belong to the Indo-Aryan physical type, and are derived largely from the same stock as the Rajputs and Dogras. Some authorities hold, however, that the Jats are of Scythian origin. Jats are divided into eastern and western. The eastern Jats inhabit the eastern districts of the Punjab and United Provinces. As a rule, only Hindus of eastern divisions are enlisted for Jat regiments. They are mainly agriculturists, and make most excellent farmers, rarely equal and never surpassed by any class of peasantry in India for industry and skill.

The foodstuffs made use of in their own homes during the important early years of life when growth is taking place are—

Bread made from wheat, juar, and other cereals.

Rabri, prepared by mixing bajra with buttermilk.

Dals and vegetables of all kinds. Rice is seldom eaten.

Milk, curds, butter, and other preparations of milk are used to a considerable extent, as the majority of families from which recruits would be obtained are able to keep their own cows and buffaloes.

Animal food enters to a very limited extent into the diet of the Jats in their own homes. Mutton, goat's flesh, and eggs are partaken of very sparingly—on an average once or twice a month. The protein element of the diet is considerably augmented by the large quantities of milk consumed even by adults.

These eastern Jats are of very fair physique, and their soldierly qualities are undoubtedly great; and though not so sturdy as some of the other races of the Punjab, their claim to be regarded as good fighting material is valid.*

The western Jats have largely taken to Mohammedanism and

* Bonarjee. " The Fighting Races of India."

Sikhism. The better classes of Sikhs are drawn from the Jat and Khattris, the finest specimens being Jat Sikhs, who possess all the virtues of the Jat of the Punjab, and many also developed by Sikhism.

Those Jats who have changed from the Hindu faith to Islamism and Sikhism have at the same time adopted the dietetic customs of their new religion. Animal food, therefore, enters much more largely into their dietaries than is the case with the eastern Jat. Large numbers of Islam converts are enlisted as Punjabi Mohammedans, as, for instance, the Kharral tribe, who are hardy, well-built, and good-looking, possessing the martial instinct to a high degree, and make very good soldiers.

The Jat Sikh is an exceptionally fine type of Asiatic, exhibiting a splendid physique, well-proportioned, and solidly built. With his manly and handsome features, his sturdy independence, self-respect, and racial pride, he is the beau ideal of an Oriental soldier. The Khalsa Sikh, or Sikh *par excellence*, is drawn from many castes, but mostly from the Punjab Jat, to whose sturdy and independent character the warlike and manly precepts of Sikhism appeal. The Jat Sikh is the truest and best embodiment of Sikhism. Jats who have adopted other religions and have not entered the fold of Khalsa, do not make nearly so good soldiers as their brothers who have taken this step.*

The dietaries of those Jat tribes who have become Mohammedans and Sikhs are considerably superior in the degree of protein metabolism they permit to those of the eastern Hindu Jats. Mohammedans in general are meat-eaters, consuming the flesh of the ordinary animals used for food in European countries, with the exception of the pig. Punjabi Mohammedans live largely on wheat, millets, maize, peas, milk in its various forms, and animal materials.

The Jat Sikh also has not attained his high position as regards physique and soldierly qualities on a diet poor in protein. Like Jats everywhere, whatever religious views they may hold, they are splendid farmers. A very large proportion are peasant proprietors, which condition insures a full sufficiency of all foodstuffs available from the land. Wheat is their staple food, but bajra, maize, and juar are also eaten during certain seasons of the year. Milk, curd, buttermilk, and butter are largely consumed.

* Bonarjee, "The Fighting Races of India."

Goat's flesh, venison, mutton, pork, game of all sorts—in fact, all animal food except beef, which is forbidden. Eggs and fish are also eaten when procurable.

The following diet gives a fair average for the daily consumption of food by the Jat Sikh. The information was obtained from native officers of a Sikh regiment.

			Protein Value.
Wheat	24 to 26 ozs.	⎫	
Dals	2 ,,	⎪	130 to 151 grms., of which over
Vegetables	4 ,,	⎬	40 per cent. is derived from an
Milk	16 ,,	⎪	animal source.
Meat	6 to 8 ,,	⎭	

When rice or millets, maize or barley, are made use of, they replace about an equal quantity of wheat; but when this is the case, usually considerably more milk is consumed. The Jats use curdled milk very largely, and buttermilk is a staple article of diet in every family.

The average dietary as outlined above is of a superior type, and would mean a high level of protein interchange. Accepting the average protein absorption to be 80 per cent., it would mean a metabolism of from 18 to 20 grammes of nitrogen daily.

Physical Development.—Jat Sikhs as a class are late of development; recruits of eighteen or nineteen years of age are often lanky, undeveloped-looking lads. As a rule they have well-shaped chests, with good expansion, and have plenty of " bone." They rapidly develop into men of powerful physique under a course of drill, gymnastics, etc., with a liberal diet.

Average height	68 to 69 inches.
,, chest girth	33 to 35 ,,
,, weight	140 to 150 lbs.

It is evident from the information collected on the influence of food on these different classes of Jats that the evidence bears out in every detail the conclusions arrived at from a similar analysis of the conditions prevailing in the several classes of Rajputs and Dogras. Contrasting tribes or sects derived from the same stock, living under identical conditions and customs, but under different dietetic standards, we are able to obtain corroboration of the views generally held by physiologists with regard to the important rôle played by protein in the nutrition of mankind, and the determining influence of a high level of nitrogenous interchange on the physique, stamina, and manly characteristics of the individuals of the races.

The facts collected and published for the guidance of recruiting officers show undoubtedly that those classes that are in a position to obtain a liberal supply of good food form the chief sources of the best fighting material, while the less well-fed classes, even though in some cases everything except diet is in their favour, are acknowledged to be inferior from a military standpoint in the necessary qualities of the soldier. We have brought forward abundant evidence on these points in considering the eastern and western Rajputs; the different classes of Dogras, particularly when discussing the effects of food on the Mians and on the lower agricultural classes, who, despite their mixed Aryan and Dravidian blood, have gradually developed into material superior in physique and stamina to the pure-blooded descendant of the old warrior stock of Rajputs; and, lastly, the effects as exhibited by the several sects of Jats, Punjabi Mohammedans, and Jat Sikhs, in each and all of whom the merits and demerits of dietaries high and low in protein respectively are very apparent and easily estimated. The evidence afforded by a study of the influence of diet on these races is entirely at variance with the views expressed by Chittenden, and can only lead to one conclusion—viz., that a sufficiently liberal degree of nitrogenous interchange is essential for the formation and development of those attributes and qualities of mind and body that are alike the pride of the soldier and the envy of inferior races.

The Sikh.

"Hardy, brave, intelligent; too slow to understand when he is beaten; obedient to discipline; attached to his officers; careless of caste prohibitions—he is unsurpassed as a soldier of the East, and takes first place as a thoroughly reliable useful soldier. The Sikh is always the same, ever genial, good-tempered, and uncomplaining; as steady under fire as he is eager for a charge. When well and sufficiently led, he is the equal of any troops in the world, and superior to any with whom he is likely to come into contact" (Falcon).

"As a soldier the Sikh displays a cool, quiet, and resolute courage, and is much less likely to lose his head in the excitement of battle than the Pathan. His passions are well under control; he knows how to keep cool and unexcited in moments of difficulty and danger. He is therefore much less liable to sudden panic than the Pathan, though he may not have the same dash and élan as the Pathan in his most warlike mood. Taken as a whole, the Sikh is one of the finest types of men to be found in Asia. Is independent without being insolent, resolute and firm in character, remarkably free from petty bias and prejudices which run rampant in a land of prejudices like India. Respects himself, and as a result commands the respect of others ; is a soldier by instinct and tradition ; regards cowardice as worse than a crime ; and with his splendid physique and well-bred ways is one of the finest of Oriental races " (Bonarjee).

Unlike the Rajputs, Dogras, or Jats, Sikhs are not the high caste descendants of the conquering Aryans. Sikhism includes within its folds all of these, but in addition many of the lower and despised classes. Thus the despised scavenging Chuhra of the Punjab, Sikhism has transformed into the soldierly Mazhabi.

The earlier Gurus of the Sikhs preached a peaceful religious life, and it was only the pressure of Mogul dominance that first turned Sikhism to thoughts of war. Har Govind, a practical and adventurous Guru, urged the necessity for a knowledge of the use of arms.

He not only permitted, but encouraged the use of flesh—except that of cows and unclean animals—as articles of diet, believing its consumption would tend to improve the strength and physique of the race. He did his utmost to instil manliness, self-reliance, and courage amongst his followers. The absence of caste drew large numbers to the Sikh fold, and many of the lower castes, but also of the higher, as Jats, Khattris, and Rajputs, embraced the Sikh faith.

After centuries of warfare and gradual consolidation, the Sikh, became united under Ranjit Singh, and overran the whole of the Punjab.

In Chapter IV. we have given the food materials and dietary of the Sikh in detail, and shown that, as in the case of the Jat Sikh, his splendid reputation and martial qualities have not been acquired on dietaries affording a low level of protein metabolism ; but, on the contrary, that the nitrogenous interchange possible from his diet scales is quite on a par with that of European soldiers.

The Sikh is a high protein-feeder ; he will eat the flesh of all the ordinary animals used as food, except the cow and buffalo. Milk in all its different preparations is very largely consumed—even the soldiers, who have to buy it out of their pay, drink up to 2 or 3 pints daily.

In connection with this the following extract from a letter written by the Adjutant of a Punjab regiment may be quoted: "As to the effects of good food, I may mention that since the regiment left Calcutta, where milk was expensive and of poor quality, and arrived in Dera Ismail Khan, where milk is cheap and good, the men have improved in health and general fitness to a great extent. As milk is the staple article of diet of the Sikh, you can easily understand that when he comes into such favourable circumstances his improvement is noticeable.'"

It is of interest to note that the Sikhs, like most Hindu tribes, marry their female children before the first menstrual period. It would not, therefore, appear that this custom has so deleterious an influence on physique as is generally thought. Infant marriage is dying out to some extent amongst the Sikhs and some other Hindu tribes.

A general idea of the physical development of the young Sikh recruit will be obtained from the following data:

Average age	.. ..	18 years.
,, height	.. ..	67$\frac{1}{2}$ inches.
,, chest girth	.. ..	33$\frac{1}{2}$ to 35$\frac{1}{2}$ inches.
,, weight	.. ..	135 to 140 lbs.

Taking the dietaries as recorded in Chapter IV., Study No. 7, and the facts given under Jat Sikhs, it may be accepted that the nitrogen metabolism of the Sikh averages from 18 to 20 grammes daily. This, for an average weight of 70 kilos, would mean the metabolism of 0·25 to 0·28 gramme of nitrogen per kilo of body weight, or more than twice the amount Chittenden and the advocates of a low protein dietary consider necessary. The Sikh is perhaps the best known of the martial tribes of the plains of India; it is therefore of interest to learn something of the dietary on which he lives. The evidence shows that, although Sikhism is composed of representatives of many different castes, some of high standing such as Rajputs, Jats, etc., and some of the despised lower classes of impure descent, such as the Chuhra and Sudra, the effect of the religious and military precepts, combined with a liberal dietary, has been to increase the physique, stamina, and soldierly qualities of those derived from the higher (a.) RAJPUT.   (b.) SIKH.   (c.) PATHAN.

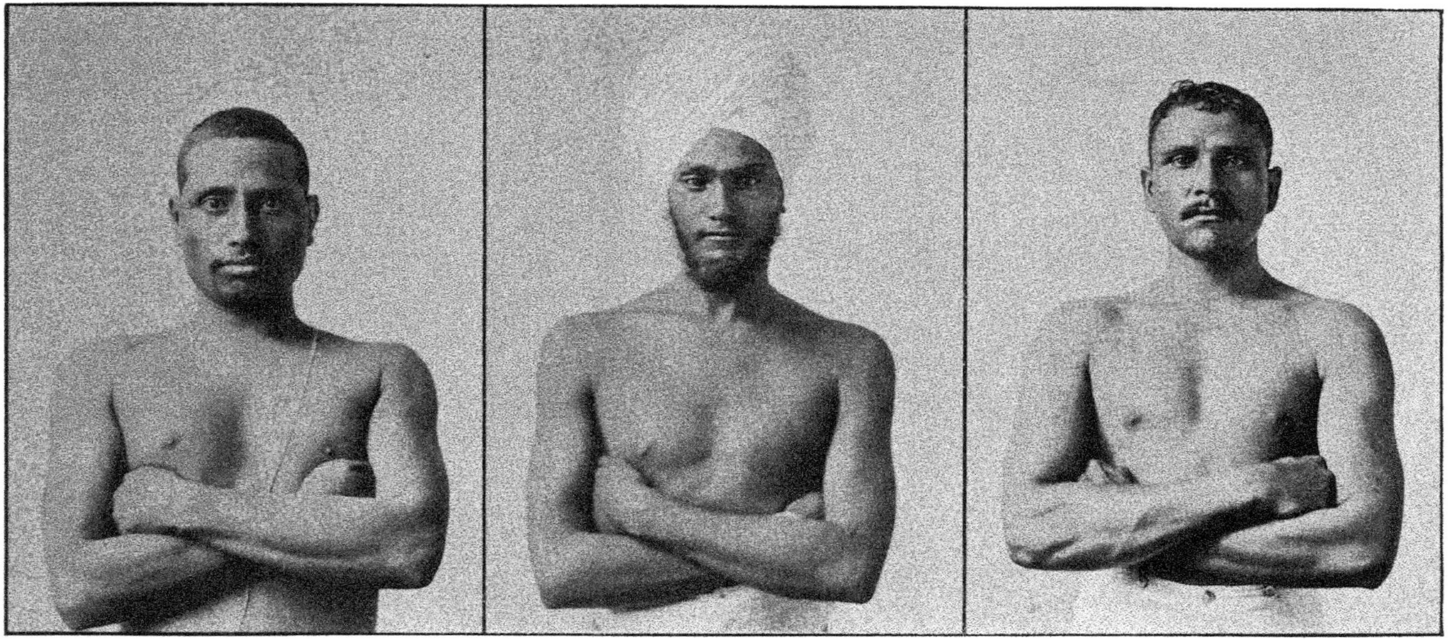

castes, and inculcate the martial spirit into those of obscure origin. The protein metabolism of the Sikh is superior to that of the other fighting tribes so far considered, and, failing any other explanation of his superior qualities, we must admit the undoubted influence of his highly nitrogenous dietary during the important early years of life—the period during which the body framework and protoplasmic tissues are being built up.

We may conclude this study of the Indo-Aryan physical type by saying that where it is possible to eliminate climatic, social, and caste influences, as in a comparison of tribes living under the same conditions, except as regards diet, there can be no doubt of the superiority, physically, morally, and socially, of those whose diet is the most liberal, and whose daily average of metabolized nitrogen reaches a high level. Having studied the effects of dietaries offering varying quantities of assimilable protein on different tribes, otherwise under similar conditions, we are more firmly than ever of the opinion that the level of protein exchange advocated by Chittenden is too low, and that a supply at least equal to that of the usually accepted standards is to the advantage of the individual and to the welfare of the race.

The Pathan.

The Pathans are given by Risley under the Turko-Iranian physical type. The Pathan himself claims to be of Jewish origin.

The different tribes are pastoral and agricultural; they possess large flocks of sheep, goats, cows, etc. Milk is highly esteemed, and the better classes live exceedingly well on a highly protein dietary of wheat, maize, milk in various forms, and large quantities of animal food. In their homes animal food is eaten daily.

They have never been accustomed to law nor settled government, and are a wild, lawless, turbulent people, to whom law and order are things to be scoffed at. Pathans are pre-eminently resolute and self-reliant. As a soldier he displays great dash and élan, but is apt to be carried away in the heat of battle. He takes a just and manly pride in himself, and considers himself superior to other races. His resolute look, upright gait, tall and muscular frame, and firm step betoken many of the qualities of the genuine man.

The Pathan is superior in physique to any of the races mentioned. As, in addition to their superior type of dietary, the

Pathan tribes come from a different stock and live mainly in the hills, we cannot make use of them in a comparison with the Rajputs, Jats, or Sikhs.

It is sufficient to point out that their splendid physique and fighting qualities have not been attained on diets permitting a low level of nitrogenous metabolism.

We may conclude this study of the effects of the level of protein metabolism on the physique and general efficiency of different tropical tribes and races by stating that the facts, as set forth in the preceding pages, afford ample proof of the all-important influence exerted by food, and particularly protein, in determining the degree of muscular development, the general physical endowment, the powers of endurance, resistance to disease, and, most important of all, the place a tribe or race has won for itself in manliness, courage, and soldierly instincts. We have no hesitation in saying that, amongst the tribes and races contrasted, the higher the level of protein interchange, the more robust and energetic, and the more manly the race.

From a practical standpoint under natural conditions, in contrast to laboratory results obtained under artificial conditions, it appears somewhat superfluous to have to insist on this point, and support what should be a foregone conclusion with a mass of evidence. But with such an eloquent appeal as that made by Chittenden for a decrease of at least 50 per cent. in the ordinary protein standard, backed up as it is by an array of such seemingly convincing arguments, it is only meet that the real facts should be brought to light before harmful measures in the feeding of large bodies of men have been adopted.

We might illustrate further the determining influences of a liberal supply of protein by a study of other races and tribes in India. Thus there are the Afridis, physically a fine type, tall, muscular, hardy, brave, proud, and self-reliant. They make ideal soldiers. The Waziris, a tribe probably of Rajput origin, who have acquired a great reputation for courage and warlike qualities. The Bajouris, physically a grand race of men, are hardy, muscular, and brave, and make good soldiers. The Baluchis are manly, frank, and strong, inured to hardships and exposure. They are a fine type of men, and have acquired a reputation for truth and fidelity. Many other sects and tribes of the Indian frontier might be made use of to show that wherever the characteristics and instincts of the soldier are to be found, there will also be present a high level of protein interchange. The different classes just mentioned are all large meat-consuming people. They are mostly pastoral, and all possess large flocks and herds. They live mainly on wheat, maize, barley, rice, milk, and animal flesh. Their country is, however, very sterile, so that the products of agriculture form a comparatively small part of the daily food.

The photographs of typical representatives of the several sects and tribes discussed will give a fair idea of the differences in physique met with amongst the inhabitants of India.

The evidence of the importance of a high level of protein metabolism is overwhelming, whatever the standpoint from which its effects be examined. Considerations of space do not permit us to do more than call attention to two important investigations carried out on this interesting subject. The first was the series of experiments with batches of soldiers to determine the food requirements for sustenance and work. The results furnished by the Committee on the "Physiological Effects of Food, Training, and Clothing on the Soldier" show that when hard marching is performed a high protein dietary is an absolute necessity.

Over periods of a fortnight of hard training the protein element was increased up to well over 200 grammes per man daily. The Committee state that these figures were undoubtedly high, but there was no evidence that they were too high.

The conclusion of the medical officers who took part in both experimental periods—with a low and high protein content of the diets—was that the best ration for service is one containing about 200 grammes of protein.

Lieutenant-Colonel Melville,[*] R.A.M.C., speaking of the results obtained during the first experimental period, states that 190 grammes of protein appeared to be ample, whilst 145 grammes was too low.

The second important series of experiments to which we wish to call attention will be found in the *Philippine Journal of Science* of February, 1911.

After a most exhaustive and brilliantly successful series of

---

[*] Melville, "Food Requirements for Sustenance and Work," *British Medical Journal*, October, 1910.

investigations to determine the influence of a restricted diet on growing dogs, Aron arrives at the following conclusions:

A growing animal which receives only sufficient food to keep its body weight constant, or to allow a slight increase, is in a condition of severe starvation.

If by a restriction of food the increase in weight is inhibited, the skeleton grows at the expense of other parts of the body, especially of the flesh.

Most of the organs retain their weight and size, while the brain grows to reach its normal weight.

The composition of the body, when at a constant weight, undergoes remarkable changes: fat is consumed more or less entirely, the quantity of protein, especially of the muscles, but not of the organs, is diminished, and a great proportion of the body tissues is replaced by water; thus this water and the increase of the skeleton together replace the body material lost.

The caloric value of 1 gramme body weight of an animal which has undergone such a process to its extreme limit may amount to only one-third of the normal value.

It is possible by supplying suitable amounts of food to maintain a dog in an emaciated condition, apparently in good health, and at the weight of a puppy, for nearly one year, while its weight at the end of the year should be three times as great. If such an animal is thereupon fed amply, it fattens and rounds out, but does not reach the size of a control animal which from the beginning has been normally fed. It is unable to make good the growth suspended by the long restriction of food.

It will be readily recognized how very closely Aron's results correspond to those obtained with dietaries poor in protein, as exemplified by the rice-eating Bengali and Ooriya. Aron experimented with dietaries deficient in energy and in all the different elements. The Bengali and Ooriya show that very similar effects are produced when—the potential energy and carbonaceous material of the diet being abundant—the protein element alone is deficient.

The Influence of Certain Substances present in the Food in Minute Quantities on the Maintenance of Nutrition.

Reference has already been made to the fact that recent lines of research point to the presence of certain substances in the food, present only in minute quantities, as being essential for the nutrition of the organism. Hill and Flack, in their work on the nutritive value of flours, have shown that foodstuffs must be regarded, not only from the standpoint of their protein content and caloric value, but also from another aspect—viz., the presence or absence of certain organic constituents which have been found to be of the very greatest importance in the growth and nutrition of the body. The researches of Funk[*] and others on the isolation of the substance contained in the polishings of rice, absence of which from the food is now generally recognized as the specific cause of beri-beri in man and polyneuritis in animals, is another example of certain materials present in the food whose importance is out of all proportion to their nitrogen content or caloric value.

It is now generally admitted that the body requires for the growth and repair of its protoplasmic tissues certain complexes or grouping of nitrogenous combinations, and that, failing a sufficient supply of these, neither growth nor nitrogenous equilibrium can be maintained, no matter how much protein may be offered in the diet. We have referred to the work done from this point of view in the first chapter of this volume. It would appear very probable that certain of these groups or combinations are provided in the organic base that Funk has isolated from rice polishings, and that Moore[†] and his co-workers have shown to be present in yeast. Such important substances would appear to be present in many other food materials in their natural state, but may be lost by certain methods of preparations—as, for instance, overmilling of cereals.

Recognizing the important bearing of these discoveries on the problems of nutrition and on the maintenance of the body in nitrogenous equilibrium, it appeared to us to be a matter of some moment to make certain that the poor physique of the Bengali was not to be attributed to the absence or insufficient supply of these essential materials in his food.

A priori the weight of evidence is strongly against such a contention or such an explanation of the poor muscular development of the Bengali. Thus, there is practically no beri-beri in Bengal, as country rice, and not the highly polished Rangoon variety, is the form in general use. Further, the fact that large quantities of dal—a substance very rich in the element lacking

---

[*] Funk, *The Journal of State Medicine*, June, 1912.
[†] Moore and others, *The Bio-Chemical Journal*, July, 1912.

in polished rice—are eaten with rice insures that an abundance of the antineurotic vitamine is provided in the food.

However, to make certain that these deductions were sound, a series of investigations were undertaken to determine what, if any, of the Bengal foodstuffs caused polyneuritis in animals, and what, if any, cured the condition.

Batches of pigeons have been fed on the different Bengal food materials for over eight months. We have nothing new to report. Shortly, the results so far in the investigations have been :

1. No Bengal foodstuff causes polyneuritis in pigeons.
2. Polished rice invariably causes the condition.
3. None of the dals in use in Bengal produce the disease.
4. Indian or country rice has no deleterious effect.
5. Polyneuritis produced by feeding on Rangoon rice is cured —(a) by feeding with Indian or country rice; (b) by feeding with alcoholic extract of rice polishings or of Indian rice; (c) by feeding with dals or the alcoholic extracts of dals.

It is evident, therefore, that the absence of the beri-beri vitamine in their dietary is not the explanation of the poor physique of the Bengalis.

Further, while there can be no doubt of the importance of these substances in growth and nutrition, the fact of the necessity of such bodies in the food is a strong argument in favour of a liberal supply of food, in order that the system may be afforded the opportunity of picking out those particular combinations which are so essential to its nutrition, and is no argument for the reduction of either the protein content or total potential value of dietaries below the generally accepted standards.

These bodies are probably of a specific nature, fulfilling certain specific functions that cannot be performed by the ordinary cleavage products of protein digestion ; but to believe, as some are inclined to do, that, because these substances have been found to be absolutely essential, therefore the protein element of the diet can be cut down to one-half or one-third of Voit's standard is to go beyond the indications warranted by the facts.

It is far more rational to believe that these vitamines are necessary in addition to the ordinary amino-acids, and that, in all probability, they can neither take the place of, nor be replaced by, the products of the tryptic digestion of proteins.

INDEX

ABDERHALDEN, experiments on horse, 8
Aboriginal tribes, 24, 28, 89
Absorbability of foods, 33; Hutchison's table of, 34; Langworthy's groups, 35
Absorbability: of fruits, Jaffa, 35; of protein of rice, 38; of tropical foodstuffs, 36
Absorption of constituents of different breads, 50
Absorption of protein: arhar dal, 66; of bajra, 55; of barley, 55; of Chittenden's subjects, 124; of juar, 55; of pulses, 59; of pulses, effects of bulk on, 64; of tropical foods, 65; uniform from identical diets, 126
Acid intoxication and acidosis, 12
Acids, monamido and diamido, 5
Afridis, characteristics of, 206
Ainus, 28
Albuminuria in Bengalis, 172
Amino-acids, 2
Ammonia: in portal vein, 6; importance of, in acidosis, 12; Schryver's views on, 13
Analysis of Indian foods, 32
Andamanese, 28
Aneurism rare in Hindus, 176
Anglo-Indian and Eurasian students: as athletes, 138; diets of, 161, 171; effects of diet, 162, 171
Army rations: caloric value of, 71; protein content and heat value of, 74
Aron: influence of a restricted diet on dogs, 208; protein absorption of rice, 38
Aryo-Dravidian physical type, 190
Atwater and Bryant, composition of foods, 31
Atwater, standards of dietaries, 71

Bajouris, characteristics of, 206
Bajra: chemical composition of, 55; protein absorption of, 55
Baluchis, characteristics of, 206

Barley: chemical composition of, 54; protein absorption of, 55
Bedouins in Arabia, meat diet, 88
Benedict: caloric value of Indian foods, 33; diets of low caloric value, 116; criticism of protein absorption of Chittenden's subjects, 124; explanation of non-uniformity of protein absorption, 125; effects of diets deficient in protein, 139; experiments on energy requirements, 146; needs of the body for food, 69; requirements of different classes, 70
Bengal infant, average weight of, 94
Bengal mother's milk: composition of, 92; amount secreted, 92
Bengal students and servants, 76; contrasted with Japanese, 77; and Chittenden's standard, 77
Bengal students: diet at college, 161; physical development of, 160, 162; as athletes, 139
Bengali: capacity for work, 166; characteristics in underfeeding, 175; classes contrasted, 181; diet of, Chittenden's misconception, 81; diet of, not ill-balanced, 82; deficiency in body fat, 98; deficiency in hæmoglobin, 158; chemical composition of blood, 157; chemical composition of urine, 156; blood-pressure of, 157; effects of underfeeding on, 159; physical development of, 164; physical endurance of, 165; life expectation of, 167; life insurance amongst, 168; protein metabolism of, 157; renal disease in, 172, 174; resisting powers to disease, 171; resistance of acute infections, 172, 174; not a soldier, 183
Bhutia: classes of, 184; development of, 185; protein metabolism of, 187; Sikhim, diet of, 86, 187; Tibetan, diet of, 86, 187
Bleaching of flour, 47
Brahmin proverb, 154

Bread, "standard," advantages claimed, 46
Browne, Crichton : criticisms of Chittenden's views, 102 ; diets, mixed and vegetable, 26
Brunton, Sir Lauder, experiments on food, 67
Buchanan, Lt.-Col., observations on physique of the Bengali, 164
Buckle, effects of an increasing supply of food, 25
Buddhism, diet allowed, 25
Bulkiness of diets, effects of, 40
Bunge, the pessimist's view of physiological research, 21
Bushmen of South Africa, diet of, 88

Caddy, Dr. A., life insurance in India, 168
Caloric value : army rations, 71 ; Indian foodstuffs, 32 ; tropical dietaries, 97
Cambridge, on the food of " Indians," 151
Campbell, Dr. Harry : conclusions regarding diet, 30 ; on the evolution of man's diet, 26
Carbohydrate group of cleavage of proteins, 5
Carbonaceous metabolism, an aspect discussed, 97
Caspari and Glassner, observations on vegetarians, 118
Cathcart, on creatinine and diet, 17
Causes of rejection for life insurance in India, 170
Chemical composition : of different parts of wheat, 45 ; of different types of flour, 46
Chittenden : criticism of his observations on students, 118 ; criticism of his observations on his three groups of subjects, 132 ; experiments on six laboratory assistants, 83 ; experiments on six dogs, 140 ; experiments on six dogs criticized, 141 ; importance of his work on nutrition, 68 ; on Folin's view of the significance of creatinine, 20 ; on the dietaries of Bengalis, 81, 178 ; on the dietetic customs of mankind, 101 ; on his own metabolism, 114 ; standard of nitrogenous metabolism, 118 ; standard of students' metabolism, 118 ; studies with three groups of subjects, 116 ; standard of nutrition exemplified in the Bengali, 77
Church, on the digestibility of the protein of pulses, 61
Cibicultural epoch in the evolution of diet, 27

Coefficient : of absorption of Indian foods, 65 ; of protein absorption, low, in certain foods, 56
Conquering races all high protein feeders, 140
Conservation of energy, law of, applied to Chittenden's experiments, 115
Convict prisons of England, diets of, 135
Cooking, effects of, on digestibility of pulses, 61
Cows, effects of feeding on diets low in protein, 142
Cramer and Krause, effects of thyroid feeding on creatinine excretion, 19
Creatinine-nitrogen and diet discussed, 15, 103
Crichton - Browne, on the effects of diets poor in protein, 133
Cultivators, Bengal, diet of, 78

Dals : chemical composition of, 57 ; different forms in use, 57 ; how used as food, 58 ; importance of, as a source of nitrogen, 58
Deficient protein, effects of, 144
Demerits of diets poor in protein, 145
Denitrifying action of intracellular enzymes, 6
Determining influence of diet on Bengalis, 181
Diamido-acids, 5
Diet : of the Sikh, 90 ; of prisons of England, effects of, 136 ; poor in protein, effects of, 113
Dietary standards, 68
Dietary studies in Bengal : students and servants, 76 ; professional class, 78 ; all classes, 78 ; students in residence, 80 ; hill-tribes, 86 ; aboriginal tribes, 88 ; infants' diet, 92
Dietary studies : in Europe and America, 70 ; in India, fighting castes, 89
Dietetic customs : of mankind, Chittenden on, 101 ; of fighting castes, 184
Digestibility of different foods, 33
Disease and underfeeding, 133
Dogras : as soldiers, 183, 198 ; characteristics of, 194 ; effects of diet on, 195 ; physical development of, 193
Dogs, experimental feeding of, 140
Dorner, on creatinine and diet, 17
Dynamic effects of a high protein diet, 123

Economy of Chittenden's standard in India, 153
Effects of diet on the fighting races of the Punjab, 201, 204, 207
Effects of low protein metabolism : on the Bengali, 178 ; on animals, 144

INDEX

Effeminacy of " Indians," 149
Efficiency and the amount of food (Spriggs), 122
Endogenous metabolism, Folin's views on, 15
Energy : a property of the nervous system, 153 ; potential of tropical dietaries, 97
Energy requirements : Benedict and Carpenter, 147 ; of Chittenden's groups of subjects, 146, 148 ; of Fletcher, 146
Errors, possible, in Chittenden's observations, 145
Esquimaux, 23
Eurasian and Anglo-Indian students : as athletes, 138 ; diets of, 161 ; physique of, 160, 162
European and Bengali infants contrasted, 94
Examination, critical, of Chittenden's results, 127
Excess excretion of waste products, 123
Exogenous metabolism, 15
Experiments, Chittenden : on three groups, 116 ; on three groups, results, 117 ; on six laboratory assistants, 83
Experiments to determine the presence or absence of the beri-beri vitamine in Bengal food-materials, 210

Fæcal carbohydrates not a true measure, 97
Fæcal nitrogen : average amount of, in Bengalis, 83 ; a true measure, 98 ; of Chittenden's subjects, 125 ; of Chittenden's assistants, 84 ; on certain vegetable diets, 57
Famine and the incidence of disease, 134
Fasting, excretion of nitrogen during, 105
Favourable results ascribed to low protein dietary, 130
Feeding on the cleavage products : of intestinal digestion, 4 ; of acid hydrolysis, 4
Fermentation, intestinal, as a cause of loss of potential energy, 97
Fischer : researches into the composition of protein, 4 ; synthesis of polypeptides, 6
Fisher, Irving, on effects of diets poor in protein, 138
Flack and Hill, the nutritive value of flours, 52
Fletcher, energy requirements of, 146
Flour : bleaching of, 47 ; false standard of millers, 49 ; wholemeal, chemical composition of, 46 ; standard, 47

Folin : deductions from urinary creatinine discussed, 103 ; significance of constancy of creatinine output, 15
Food : its functions, 23, 96 ; of Brahmins, 150
Food-materials of India, absorption of, 65
Food requirements of different classes, 70
Foods : American and European, analyses of, 32 ; Indian, analyses of, 32
France, prison diets of, 137
Fuegians, diet of, 23
Funk, isolation of beri-beri vitamine, 52, 209

Gaols of Bengal : dietaries of, 81 ; dietaries ill-balanced, 82
Gaols of India, absorption of protein of pulses, 62
Gautier, Dr., on prison diets of France, 137
Glycosuria in Bengalis, 172
Goodfellow, on the nutritive value of Hovis bread, 45
Graham flour, absorption of constituents of, 50
Granular kidney in different races in India, 177
Grinding-stones in India, 45

Haecker, on feeding cows on low protein diets, 144
Hagemann, experiments on dogs, 140
Hale, on the effects of nitrites in flour, 48
Halliburton, on the effects of nitrites in flour, 47
Hamill and Schryver, observations on scientists, 118
Hansen and Henriques, experiments on rats, 3
Harcourt, absorption of protein of maize, 53
Harden, effects of bleaching on flours, 48
Hill and Flack, the nutritive value of flours, 52
Hill-tribes of Bengal, characteristics of, 184
Hindus : acute infection in, 175 ; atheroma and granular kidney in, 177 ; diet of, 24 ; mortality rates of, 167 ; renal disease in, 174
Hoesslin, effects of underfeeding on the blood, 159
Hofman, protein absorption of vegetable diets, 41
Hogs, effects of a low protein diet on, 143, 144
Hoogenhuyze and Verploegh, on creatinine excretion, 17

Hopkins : on the elaboration of suprarenal secretion, 8 ; and Willcock, on the protein of maize, 7
Hutchison : criticism of Chittenden's views, 101 ; degrees of health, 153 ; on the effects of diets poor in protein, 133 ; on the merits of a high protein standard, 123 ; table of coefficients of absorption of food constituents, 34 ; vegetable protein absorption, 42

Ill-balanced dietaries of Bengal gaols, 82
Ill-effects of low protein dietaries, 146
Improvers, effects of, on weak wheats, 48
India, dietary studies in : students and servants, 76 ; professional class, 78 ; all classes of Bengalis, 78 ; different classes of students, 85 ; hill-tribes of Bengal, 86 ; aboriginal tribes of Chota Nagpur, 88 ; fighting castes, Sikh, 89 ; Bengali mother's milk and infant's food, 92
Indian corn or maize as a food, 52
Indian corn, protein absorption of, 53
Indian dandywallahs v. Japanese jinricksha men, 75
Indian food-materials : absorbability of, 65 ; analyses of, 32
Indian v. Anglo-Indian students as athletes, 139
Indo-Aryan physical type, 189 ; influence of diet on, 205
Influence : of certain substances (vitamines) on nutrition, 208 ; of diet on physique of hill-tribes, 187 ; of high protein metabolism on the fighting races of India, 206
Insufficient protein, effects of, 131
Insurance, life, and the Bengali, 168
Intestinal fermentation and loss of potential energy, 98
Irregularity of Chittenden's figures for protein absorption, 127

Jaffa, protein absorption of fruits, 35
Jägerroos, experiments with dogs, 140
Japan, dietary studies in, 72
Japanese Navy, effects of a change of diet, 76
Jat Sikh, diet of, and physique of, 200
Jats, classes of, and diet of, 199
Jinricksha man, dietary study with, 74
Juar : chemical composition of, 55 ; protein absorption of, 55

Kaufmann and Murlin, experiments with gelatin, 7
Kellogg, effects of a low protein dietary, 179
Kidney disease in Bengal, 172, 173

Kossel, researches on protein, 4
Krause and Cramer, thyroid feeding and creatinine excretion, 19
Kristeller and Levene, investigations on creatinine, 18
Kuhne, the action of trypsin, 3

Landois, weight for height rule, 165
Langworthy, absorption of foods, 35
Leathes, explanation of acid and tryptic hydrolysis, 4
Leguminosæ, foods derived from, 57
Leowi, feeding with products of tryptic digestion, 3
Levene and Kristeller, researches on creatinine, 18
Liebig : distinction between animals and plants, 2 ; view of nitrogenous metabolism, 15
Livingstone, diets of tribes of Central Africa, 17
Local Government Reports : on bleaching of flour, 47 ; on use of improvers, 48
Loeser : observations on Transvaal miners, 148 ; statement regarding diet of Chittenden's soldier group, 148
Lower limits of nitrogenous equilibrium, 106
Lymphocytosis and a diet of raw meat, 134

Macaulay, characteristics of the Bengali, 154
Maize : as a food, Woods on, 54 ; protein content and protein absorption, 53
Malnutrition of renal epithelium accompanying chronic underfeeding, 123
Margin of safety (Rubner), 113
Mellanby, researches on creatinine, 17
Melville, Lt.-Col., R.A.M.C., on protein requirements, 207
Michaud, effects of feeding dogs on dog's flesh, 7
Middle classes of Bengal, diet of, 79
Milk, Bengali mother's : chemical composition of, 92 ; quantity secreted daily, 93
Minimum, physiological, of protein metabolism, 106
Minimum protein diet, how obtained, 12
Mixed form of dietary amongst precibiculturists, 88
Mohammedans : acute infectious diseases of, 175 ; atheroma and granular kidney of, 177 ; mortality rates of, 167 ; renal disease of, 174
Monamido-acids, 5
Montesquieu, on the effeminacy of " Indians," 149

INDEX

Mongolo-Dravidian physical type, 188
Mongoloid physical type, 189
Moore, isolation of vitamine from yeast, 209
Mullick, on the effects of underfeeding of students, 135
Mundas, diet of, 88
Munk, experiments on dogs, 140
Murlin and Kaufmann, experiments with gelatin, 7

Nencki, on the amount of ammonia in portal blood, 11
Nepalese: diets of, 86; classes of, 184; contrasted with their neighbours, 186; development of, 186; nitrogenous metabolism of, 188
Nietzsche, on the effects of a great error in diet, 134
Nitrites as bleachers of flour, effects of, 47
Nitrogen: excretion of, during muscle work, 109; of urine not a true measure of protein metabolism, 119
Nitrogenous metabolism: level of, in different classes of Bengalis, 87, 118; lower limits of, 106; standard fixed by Chittenden, 118; students in America, 119; ideal level of, 164
Nutrition, its problem, 155

Organic bases present in foods (vitamines), 52, 209
Orme, characteristics of "Indians," 149
Oshima, absorption of protein: of rice, 38; of pulses, 59
Oshima, dietary studies: in Japan, 72; with jinricksha man, 74
Oshima, rice not the only food of the Japanese, 73

Pampas, Indians of, 23
"Patents," finest flour, chemical composition of, 46
Pathan, characteristics and dietary of, 205
Paton: on creatinine and diet, 17; on the rôle of protein in muscle work, 108
Pators, diet of, 88
Peptides, Fischer on their derivation, 4
Pflüger's views on nitrogenous metabolism, 15
Physique to be expected with Chittenden's standard, 131, 178
Pig, experimental feeding of, 143
Potential energy, loss of, in urine and fæces, 96
Prausnitz, on the absorption of protein of pulses, 59
Precibicultural epoch in the evolution of man's diet, 27

Precibiculturists and a mixed form of alimentation, 88
Precookery, 27
Pre-mortal rise in nitrogen excretion, 106
Prison dietaries: in France, 137; in Scotland, 136
Protein: a nerve food, 153; as a source of energy for muscle work, 108; of dietaries of Bengali and Eurasian students, 162
Protein absorption of Chittenden's subjects, 124
Protein material: its importance, 1; from animal and vegetable kingdoms contrasted, 8
Protein metabolism: ideal level of, 164; of different tribes in Bengal, 87, 89; of jinrickshaman in Japan, 75; of students in America, 119; of students and servants in Bengal, 76; Sikh, 91; standard recommended by Chittenden, 118; lower limits of, 106
Protein requirements of mankind, 96
Protein-poor dietaries, observations by different observers, 114
Pulses: importance of, as a food in India, 58; protein absorption, investigations, 59
Pyrimidine group in the cleavage of proteins, 5
Pyrrol group, 5

Races of the Gangetic Plain, 188
Rajputs: as soldiers, 183; classes of, 191; influence of diet on, 192; physique of, 193
Rations, army, caloric value of, 71
Recruits, rejection of, and underfeeding, 123
Renal disease in Bengal, 173, 174
Renal epithelium, malnutrition of, 172
Rice: absorption of the protein element, 38; as the staple food of parts of India, 37; classes of, 37
Rice diet: bulkiness of, 38; not the principal food of India, 151; the cause of effeminacy, 150
Richter, absorption of protein of pulses, 59
Risley, the people of India, 181, 189
Roberts, food customs of mankind, importance of, 102
Rogers: analysis of post-mortem records, 173; effects of diet on mortality, 176
Rosenheim, experiments on dogs, 140
Rowntree, effects of underfeeding, 123
Rubner, absorption of protein: of maize, 53; of pulses, 59
Rubner, margin of safety, 113
Russell, strength and diet, 68

Sawanis, diet of, 88
Schryver, rôle of ammonia in metabolism, 13
Schutzenberg, composition of protein, 4
Scotch prisoners, diet of, 136
Scrafton on the food of "Indians," 151
Sexual excess in India, 180
Shaffer, excretion of creatinine, 17
Shutt, experimental feeding of hogs, 143
Sikh : as a soldier, 184, 202 ; effects of diet and Sikhism on, 204 ; dietaries of, 90, 203 ; nitrogenous metabolism of, 91 ; not a vegetarian, 91 ; physique of, 204
Sikh, Jat : as a soldier, 200 ; physique of, 201
Sivén, exp riments with diets poor in nitrogen, 113
Skinner, experimental feeding of hogs, 144
Snyder : experiments with preparations of wheat, 50 ; on the protein absorption of pulses, 59
Soldier group of Chittenden, Loeser on their diet, 148
Solitary cells for prisoners under observation, 132
Spriggs, quantity of food necessary for efficiency, 122
"Standard" bread : advantages claimed for, 46
Standard dietaries, table of, 69
Standard dietary, 68
Starvation and the nitrogen requirements, 105
Stewart, on the metabolism of proteins, 110
Strachey : on Indian foodstuffs, 151 ; on the characteristics of the Bengali, 154
Strength, increase of, in Chittenden's subjects, 124
Strumpell, the effects of cooking on protein absorption, 66
Students, Chittenden's observations on, 119
Studies, dietary : in Europe and America, 70 ; in Bengal, 76
Sudra, caste or class of, 194
Sulphur-carrying group in the cleavage of proteins, 5
Summary of criticisms of Chittenden's conclusions, 132

Tibetan Bhutias : diet of, 86, 187 ; physique of, 185
Tiegel, on the food of the Japanese, 75
Todas : diet of, 88 ; ignorance of salt, 88
Torulin of yeast (Moore), 209
Types, physical : of India, 187 ; effects of diet on, 188

Underfeeding, effects : on Bengali, 159 ; on blood, 159 ; of, in disease, 133
Uraons, diet of, 88
Urinary nitrogen : as a measure of protein metabolism, 119, 132 ; of Chittenden's subjects, 129
Urine of Bengalis, chemical composition of, 156

Vaisiya, caste of, 194
Vedas, hymns in Sanskrit language, 193
Veddahs of Ceylon, 28
Vegetarian couple, observations on, 118
Vegetarianism in India and Japan, 72
Verploegh, creatinine metabolism, 17
Verworn, the metabolism of proteins, 1
Vitamine of beri-beri (Funk), 52, 209
Voit, standard of protein : in diet, 101 ; contrasted with Chittenden's students, 121
V. Noorden : high protein feeding and health, 124 ; table giving experiments with diets poor in protein, 114 ; table showing results of Chittenden's experiments, 117 ; working man's demand for protein, 100

Wait, absorption of protein of pulses, 59
Waller, the state of nutrition, 153
Waste products, excess in the urine, 123
Waziris, characteristics of, 206
Weber, creatinine and muscular activity, 20
Weight of European and Bengali infant, 94
Weir-Mitchell treatment and high feeding, 134
Wheat : protein content and protein absorption, 43 ; protein absorption in India, 44
Wheat-meal, composition of, 46
Willcock and Hopkins, experiments with zein, 7
Winter, life insurance in India, 168
Woodruff, Major, U.S.A. : actinic rays, effects of, 180 ; on diets in the tropics, 24
Woods, on maize as a food, 54
Work : demand for protein in severe, 100 ; source of energy in, 107

Zieman, on the influence of diet on the tribes of tropical Africa, 138

From
Mr. Edward Arnold's List
of
Medical Books.

WORKS BY DR. ROBERT HUTCHISON.

FOOD AND THE PRINCIPLES OF DIETETICS.

By ROBERT HUTCHISON, M.D. Edin., F.R.C.P., Physician to the London Hospital, and Assistant Physician to the Hospital for Sick Children, Great Ormond Street. New and Revised Edition, 1911. xx + 615 pages, with Illustrations. 16s. net.

The *British Medical Journal* says:
(First Edition.) "Accepted as the leading work amongst English text-books on Dietetics."

(Latest Edition.) "The best work of its kind which has been published in recent years by any one in this country."

LECTURES ON DISEASES OF CHILDREN.

Second Edition, revised and enlarged. xii + 426 pages, with 64 Plates and 13 Diagrams. Crown 8vo., cloth, 8s. 6d. net.

"The whole of the book has been revised, and may be commended as a safe and convenient guide to the practitioner."—*Lancet.*

"In the second revised edition fresh chapters have been inserted. Each of these additions enhances the value and usefulness of the work. Dr. Hutchison possesses the happy gift of stating the main essentials of each complaint in a plain and lucid manner."—*British Medical Journal.*

LONDON: EDWARD ARNOLD, 41 & 43 MADDOX STREET, W.

THIRD EDITION, REVISED AND ENLARGED.

THE DIAGNOSIS OF NERVOUS DISEASES.

By PURVES STEWART, M.A., M.D. Edin., F.R.C.P., Physician to Out-Patients at the Westminster Hospital; Joint Lecturer on Medicine in the Medical School; Physician to the West End Hospital for Nervous Diseases, and to the Royal National Orthopædic Hospital; Consulting Physician to the Central London Throat Hospital. 476 pages, with 208 Illustrations from Original Diagrams and Clinical Photographs. 15s. net.

"To practitioners unable to profit by post-graduate study, the careful descriptions, illustrated by the author's photographs, of the various methods of clinical investigation, the correct methods of eliciting the many superficial and deep reflexes, of performing lumbar puncture, of making an electro-diagnosis, and so on, and the significance of these phenomena in disease, will be simply invaluable. The whole book, which is beautifully illustrated and most carefully indexed, though in no way intended to replace the larger text-books already in use, will be found to be a most valuable supplement which we cannot too strongly commend to practitioners and students."—*British Medical Journal.*

*** *Translations of this work in German and French (from the Second Edition), have recently been published.*

A SYSTEM OF CLINICAL MEDICINE

DEALING WITH THE DIAGNOSIS, PROGNOSIS, AND TREATMENT OF DISEASE.

By the late THOMAS DIXON SAVILL, M.D. Lond. Third Edition, Revised by AGNES SAVILL, M.A., M.D. Glas., and others. xxviii + 964 pages. With 4 Coloured Plates and 172 other Illustrations. 8vo., 25s. net.

"In writing 'A System of Clinical Medicine' Dr. Savill has adopted a plan which we believe will be found of great assistance both to students and to practitioners. He has approached the subject from the standpoint of symptomatology. . . . This scheme has been admirably carried out. . . . A very useful and practical work. . . . At the end of the volume are a large number of useful formulæ for prescriptions. . . . We have formed a high opinion of Dr. Savill's work; we wish it the success that it deserves."—*Lancet.*

PRACTICAL ANATOMY.

THE STUDENT'S DISSECTING MANUAL.

By F. G. PARSONS, F.R.C.S. Eng., Lecturer on Anatomy at St. Thomas's Hospital and at the London School of Medicine for Women; Examiner for the Fellowship of the Royal College of Surgeons of England; formerly Hunterian Professor at the College of Surgeons; Examiner at the Universities of Cambridge, Aberdeen, London, and Birmingham, etc.; and WILLIAM WRIGHT, M.B., D.Sc., F.R.C.S. Eng., Lecturer on Anatomy at the London Hospital; Examiner at the Royal College of Surgeons of England, and at the Universities of London and Bristol; formerly Hunterian Professor to the Royal College of Surgeons of England.

In Two Volumes. With many Illustrations. Large crown 8vo. Price per volume, 8s. 6d. net.

The object of the authors has been to provide a book which shall contain all those anatomical facts which it is essential for a medical student to know, omitting the anatomical knowledge which is not necessary for the student.

The authors recognize that, allowing for a reasonable amount of holidays, medical students have only some fifteen months in which to learn the anatomy of the body, and it is unreasonable to expect that they will be able to exercise very just discrimination in settling for themselves what they should really learn and what they may safely leave out. In this connection the authors have been fortunate in obtaining the advice of teachers, physicians, surgeons, and specialists of acknowledged reputation.

Practical Physiology. By M. S. PEMBREY, M.A., M.D.; A. P. BEDDARD, M.A., M.D.; J. S. EDKINS, M.A., M.B. L. HILL, M.B., F.R.S.; J. J. R. MACLEOD, M.B. Third (Revised) Edition. 14s. net.

"It seems invidious in a book which is the joint work of several authors to single out any part where all is well and accurately rendered in accordance with the most recent advances in science; we can, however, assure the student that, armed with the knowledge that he will acquire by sedulously following the scheme of work laid down for him in orderly fashion in addition to his usual studies, he will be well equipped for the examination of patients and the diagnosis of disease. The application of the facts that are given, if thoroughly understood, will be the work of his life in the sick-room, and will distinguish him from the (sometimes misnamed) practical but imperfectly educated man."—*Lancet.*

Recent Advances in Physiology and Bio-Chemistry.

By LEONARD HILL, M.B.; BENJAMIN MOORE, M.A., D.Sc; J. J. R. MACLEOD, M.B.; M. S. PEMBREY, M.A., M.D.; and A. P. BEDDARD, M.A., M.D. 752 pages. 18s. net.

"This excellent work, which is admirably produced, may be recommended to all medical men who desire to acquaint themselves with the latest views upon the subjects mentioned above. Moreover, the book should be carefully studied by all senior students in physiology who intend to present themselves for any of the higher examinations."—*Practitioner.*

Further Advances in Physiology. Edited by Dr. LEONARD HILL. With contributions by Experts in various branches. 448 pages. 15s. net.

"There can be little doubt that in 'Further Advances in Physiology' Dr. Leonard Hill and his coadjutors have produced a book which will be of great use not only to advanced students of physiology, but to the clinician who wishes to interpret his results in the light of modern physiology."—*British Medical Journal.*

Applied Physiology. By ROBERT HUTCHISON, M.D. Edin., F.R.C.P., Physician to the London Hospital and to the Hospital for Sick Children, Great Ormond Street. 7s. 6d. net.

Physiology of the Special Senses. By M. GREENWOOD, Jun., M.R.C.S., L.R.C.P., F.S.S., Director of the London Hospital Statistical Department; Senior Demonstrator of Physiology in the London Hospital Medical College; Examiner in Physiology to the University of St. Andrews. viii + 239 pages. 8s. 6d. net.

The Physiological Action of Drugs. An Introduction to Practical Pharmacology. By M. S. PEMBREY, M.A., M.D., Lecturer on Physiology, Guy's Hospital; and C. D. F. PHILLIPS, M.D., LL.D. With 68 Diagrams and Tracings. Demy 8vo., cloth, 4s. 6d. net.

Human Embryology and Morphology. By ARTHUR KEITH, M.D. Aberd., F.R.C.S. Eng., Conservator of the Royal College of Surgeons. xii + 402 pages. Second Edition. 12s. 6d. net.

A Text-Book of Medical Treatment. Alphabetically Arranged. By WILLIAM CALWELL, M.A., M.D., Physician, Royal Victoria Hospital, Belfast; University Clinical Lecturer on Medicine, Queen's University, Belfast. iv + 632 pages. Royal 8vo., 16s. net.

A Pocket-Book of Treatment. By RALPH WINNINGTON LEFTWICH, M.D. viii + 348 pages. Flexible binding, with wallet flap, 6s. net.

The Treatment of Diseases of the Skin. By W. K. SIBLEY, M.A., M.D., B.C. Camb., M.R.C.P. Lond., M.R.C.S. Eng., Physician to St. John's Hospital for Diseases of the Skin, London. With Illustrations from Original Photographs. 5s. net.

Glaucoma. An Inquiry into the Physiology and Pathology of the Intra-Ocular Pressure. By THOMSON HENDERSON, M.D. Edin., Surgeon, Nottingham and Midland Eye Infirmary. Illustrated. 10s. 6d. net.

A Guide to the Diseases of the Nose and Throat, and their Treatment. By CHARLES A. PARKER, F.R.C.S. Edin., Surgeon to the Throat Hospital, Golden Square, W. xii + 624 pages. With 254 Illustrations. 18s. net.

A Handbook of Skin Diseases and their Treatment. By ARTHUR WHITFIELD, M.D. Lond., F.R.C.P., Professor of Dermatology at King's College; Physician to the Skin Departments, King's College and the Great Northern Central Hospitals. xii + 320 pages With Illustrations. 8s. 6d. net.

The House-Surgeon's Vade-Mecum. By RUSSELL
HOWARD, M.B., M.S., F.R.C.S., Surgeon to the Poplar Hospital; Assistant Surgeon to the London Hospital. With 142 Illustrations. viii+516 pages. 7s. 6d. net.

Contributions to Abdominal Surgery. By HAROLD
LESLIE BARNARD, M.S. F.R.C.S., Late Assistant Surgeon, London Hospital. xix+391 pages. Illustrated. Price 15s. net.

Movable Kidney : its Pathology, Symptoms, and
Treatment. By H. W. WILSON, M.B., B.S. Lond., F.R.C.S. Eng., Demonstrator of Anatomy, St. Bartholomew's Hospital; and C. M. HINDS HOWELL, M.A., M.B., M.R.C.P. Lond., Junior Demonstrator of Physiology, St. Bartholomew's Hospital. 4s. 6d. net.

Fractures and Separated Epiphyses. By A. J.
WALTON, M.S., F.R.C.S., L.R.C.P., Surgical Registrar, London Hospital. 312 pages. 100 Illustrations. 10s. 6d. net.

The Chemical Investigation of Gastric and In-
testinal Diseases by the Aid of Test Meals. By VAUGHAN HARLEY, M.D. Edin., M.R.C.P., F.C.S., Professor of Pathological Chemistry, University College, London ; and FRANCIS GOODBODY, M.D. Dubl., M.R.C.P., Assistant Professor of Pathological Chemistry, University College, London. 8s. 6d. net.

The Influence of Alcohol and other Drugs on
Fatigue. By W. H. RIVERS, M.D., F.R.C.P., F.R.S., Lecturer on Physiological and Experimental Psychology at Cambridge University. 6s. net.

Modern Theories of Diet, and their Bearing upon
Practical Dietetics. By A. BRYCE, M.D., D.P.H. (Camb.). 7s. 6d. net.

The Chemical Basis of Pharmacology. An Intro-
duction to Pharmaco-dynamics Based on the Study of the Carbon Compounds. By FRANCIS FRANCIS, D.Sc., Ph.D., Professor of Chemistry, University College, Bristol ; and J. M. FORTESCUE-BRICKDALE, M.A., M.D. Oxon. 384 pages. 14s. net.

A Manual of Pharmacology. By WALTER E.
DIXON, M.A., M.D., B.Sc. Lond., D.P.H. Camb., Professor of Materia Medica and Pathology, King's College, London; Examiner in Pharmacology n the Universities of Cambridge and Glasgow. Demy 8vo., 15s. net.

Military Hygiene and Sanitation. By Col. C. H.
MELVILLE, M.B. Edin., D.P.H., R.A.M.C., Professor of Hygiene, Royal Army Medical College. 418 pages. 12s. 6d. net.

The Sanitary Officer's Handbook of Practical
Hygiene. By Major C. F. WANHILL, R.A.M.C., Assistant Professor of Hygiene, Royal Army Medical College ; and Major W. W. O. BEVERIDGE, D.S.O., R.A.M.C., Analyst to the Army Medical Advisory Board. Interleaved with blank pages for notes. Crown 8vo., 5s. net

BOOKS FOR NURSES.

Surgical Nursing and the Principles of Surgery for
Nurses. By RUSSELL HOWARD, M.B., M.S., F.R.C.S., Assistant Surgeon to the London Hospital and Lecturer on Surgical Nursing to the Probationers of the London Hospital. Crown 8vo., with Illustrations, 6s.

Midwifery for Nurses. By HENRY RUSSELL
ANDREWS, M.D., B.Sc. Lond., M.R.C.P. Lond., Assistant Obstetric Physician to the London Hospital; Examiner to the Central Midwives Board. New Edition. 4s. 6d. net.

INTERNATIONAL MEDICAL MONOGRAPHS.

GENERAL EDITORS:

LEONARD HILL, M.B., F.R.S.,
Lecturer on Physiology, London Hospital Medical School

AND

WILLIAM BULLOCH, M.D.,
Bacteriologist and Lecturer on Bacteriology and General Pathology, London Hospital.

IN this series, under the general editorial supervision of Dr. Leonard Hill and Dr. William Bulloch, will be published at short intervals Monographs dealing with subjects of exceptional interest and importance, each by a leading authority, who has made a special study of the particular subject.

Readers interested in any special branch of medical science, or who are following the rapid progress of knowledge in some new phase of research will, it is hoped, find in a concise form the results of the leading investigators throughout the world. The practising physician also will find the volumes of great value, special attention being given to the practical application of the results of scientific research to the treatment of disease.

On the following pages is given a list of the volumes just published and those which it is hoped will be ready shortly; new Monographs will be added from time to time as occasion arises.

Each work can be obtained separately. Further particulars of any of the volumes in the International Medical Monograph Series, together with specimen pages, will be sent on request by the Publisher.

INTERNATIONAL MEDICAL MONOGRAPHS.

THE MECHANICAL FACTORS OF DIGESTION.

By WALTER B. CANNON, A.M., M.D., George Higginson Professor of Physiology, Harvard University. xii + 227 pages, cloth, illustrated. 10s. 6d. net.

SYPHILIS:

A SYSTEMATIC ACCOUNT OF SYPHILIS FROM THE MODERN STANDPOINT.

By JAMES MCINTOSH, M.D. Aberd., Grocers' Research Scholar; and PAUL FILDES, M.B., B.C. Camb., Assistant to the Bacteriologist of the London Hospital. xvi + 228 pages, illustrated with 8 Full-page Plates and 5 Diagrams, cloth. 10s. 6d. net.

BLOODVESSEL SURGERY AND ITS APPLICATIONS.

By CHARLES CLAUDE GUTHRIE, M.D., Ph.D., Professor of Physiology and Pharmacology, University of Pittsburgh, etc. xii + 350 pages, 158 Illustrations, cloth. 14s. net.

CAISSON DISEASE AND DIVER'S PALSY.

THE ILLNESS OF WORKERS IN COMPRESSED AIR.

By LEONARD HILL, M.B., F.R.S., Lecturer on Physiology, London Hospital. 10s. 6d. net.

INTERNATIONAL MEDICAL MONOGRAPHS

LEAD POISONING AND LEAD ABSORPTION:
THE SYMPTOMS, PATHOLOGY AND PREVENTION, WITH SPECIAL REFERENCE TO THEIR INDUSTRIAL ORIGIN AND AN ACCOUNT OF THE PRINCIPAL PROCESSES INVOLVING RISK.

By THOMAS M. LEGGE, M.D. Oxon., D.P.H. Cantab., H.M. Medical Inspector of Factories; Member of the Committee on Compensation for Industrial Diseases; Lecturer on Factory Hygiene, University of Manchester; and KENNETH W. GOADBY, D.P.H. Cantab., Pathologist and Lecturer on Bacteriology, National Dental Hospital.

THE PROTEIN ELEMENT IN NUTRITION.

By Major D. McCAY, M.B., B.CH., B.A.O., M.R.C.P. Lond., I.M.S., Professor of Physiology, Medical College, Calcutta; Examiner in Physiology, Calcutta and Punjab University.

SHOCK:
THE PATHOLOGICAL PHYSIOLOGY OF SOME MODES OF DYING.

By YANDELL HENDERSON, PH.D., Professor of Physiology, Yale University.

THE CARRIER PROBLEM IN INFECTIOUS DISEASE.
WITH PARTICULAR REFERENCE TO
ENTERIC FEVER, DIPHTHERIA, CEREBRO-SPINAL MENINGITIS, BACILLARY DYSENTERY AND CHOLERA.

By J. C. G. LEDINGHAM, D.Sc., M.B., M.A., Chief Bacteriologist, Lister Institute of Preventive Medicine, London; and G. F. PETRIE, M.D., Lister Institute of Preventive Medicine, London.

LONDON: EDWARD ARNOLD, 41 & 43 MADDOX STREET W.

RETURN TO the circulation desk of any
University of California Library

or to the

NORTHERN REGIONAL LIBRARY FACILITY
Bldg. 400, Richmond Field Station
University of California
Richmond, CA 94804-4698

ALL BOOKS MAY BE RECALLED AFTER 7 DAYS

- 2-month loans may be renewed by calling
  (510) 642-6753
- 1-year loans may be recharged by bringing
  books to NRLF
- Renewals and recharges may be made
  4 days prior to due date

Lightning Source UK Ltd.
Milton Keynes UK
UKHW022010071218
333658UK00009B/446/P